DE.

MW00423103

HOW MODERN MEDICINE HAS BETRAYED US ALL

By Stephen D. Herman, M. D., DABR

"A set of lies agreed upon" - Napoleon 1798

Published by WOLF BANE publishing company
2009

To Jeannie & Kenny
From the beginning to the end

PROLOGUE

Merck Pharmaceuticals recent debacle over the drug Vioxx is estimated to have killed 60 thousand people and caused 150 thousand heart attacks.

The malfeasance associated with this scandal is, unfortunately, only the very tip of the iceberg. The full story demonstrates a ubiquitous practice of the entire medical industry of promoting useless and toxic drugs for profit. Even worse, this same industry carefully prevents the availability of useful and safe drugs. The result is more than 600,000 unnecessary deaths each year in the U.S. and an astounding 3 million worldwide.

No person should ever visit a doctor without having read this book! No person should take any medication without having read this book! Above all, no person should take their child to a doctor without having read this book!

In this book I intend to present obvious and compelling truths in a straight forward manner, understandable to the average person and perhaps even understandable to the medical profession. This book is not intended as an academic text but as an easily comprehensible exposition based on data presented in major peer reviewed journals.

The revelations in this book may be difficult to believe-but are true nevertheless.

The revelations in this book are of vital concern to everyone.

The revelations in this book should make you angry.

The revelations in this book may save your life.

TABLE OF CONTENTS

An introduction into the patterns of drug industry malfeasance and the complicity of the medical establishment. A preparation for an epiphany of the unthinkable reality that, chapter by chapter, emerges from the dismantling of the corrupt edifice of modern pharmaceutical medicine.

Begins debunking the fictional hypotheses which are used to convince us, that thanks to the pharmaceutical industry, we are living longer and healthier lives. This fiction is unraveled along with the preposterous claim of "turning the tide" against cancer.

We delve deeper into the methodology underlying our acceptance of useless and toxic drugs. Particularly in reference to the marketers emphasis on the prevention of heart disease and stroke.

The first and most important false hypothesis underlying the modern treatment of heart disease is the cholesterol myth. This myth is dismantled with overwhelming data. We are now prepared for the ushering in of the greatest corporate bonanza in history -- Lipitor

The next false premise purporting to effectively treat heart disease is the use of statin drugs (Lipitor). By now we must be getting a glimmer of the unthinkable truth. The data doesn't lie. The toxicity is real and not one life has been saved.

A frightening exposition of the terrible toll in death and adverse events we suffer from the prescription of drugs we take with the" risk/benefit" ratio being all risk.

The hallowed aspirin a day to ward off the always eminent heart attack or stroke. Another pillar of salt washed away with clear and incontrovertible data. One additional step toward the epiphany that the drugs that we are told are saving us are actually killing us.

Again we examine a price to be paid for the acceptance, without reservation, of a useless drug by more than fifty million souls. Another hidden death toll.

A revelation about what may be the single most egregious and costly false proposition permeating all of modern medicine - - the fiction that oxygen free - radicals are toxic and that vitamins and antioxidants are good for you. This chapter thoroughly debunks this myth, which is the basis for an unprecedented marketing bonanza, from the doctor's office to the supermarket. This myth may well be the single most costly in terms of human lives and that leads us directly into the most important chapter of this book.

The story within the story begins here. It is about a doctor who wouldn't accept flawed science when the specter of AIDS began killing on a massive scale. He knew that there had to be a better way. And this unleashed a whirlwind. This chapter begins the journey of Dr. D and an AIDS patient named Scotty and ultimately takes us to Africa and the solution to AIDS.

The story of the development of a better way - - a way that the world did not want. A safe and effective technology - now proven - but a threat to the massive tower of deception that controls the world of medicine and the world of AIDS.

This chapter returns us to the process of deconstructing the tower of deception. It continues the revelation of the failure of so-called "blockbuster" medicines starting with the anxiety and depression drugs which have turned millions of Americans into unwitting junkies.

Drugs for the treatment of arthritis and related aches and pains account for more than one third of the pharmaceutical dollar - that is more than two hundred billion dollars yearly. And now the burgeoning market for bone density treatment is being worked for all its worth. What are we getting for our joint pain-- blockbusters or bone busters?

Sometimes it is difficult to pee and sometimes it's too easy to pee, and there is money to be made in both instances. Show me a man with a large prostate whose urologist hasn't given him Avodart and Flomax and I'll show you a man without a urologist. Show me a woman with a hyperactive bladder and I'll show you a woman with pills called Vesicare (or Detrol) and a hyperactive bladder.

Yes there are some good drugs - usually older ones - but there are lots of bad drugs and there are some really bad drugs. Really good drugs are practically non- existent and thus the drug companies continue to chase the failures. We will look at the top 20 hit parade of drugs - can I even keep my own family away from them?

The story of a billion dollar scam for a ten cent medicine to save us from the Avian flu - 60% death rate without Tamiflu ---70% death rate with the billion dollar miracle Tamiflu. Ten billion for a totally useless flu vaccine --an   introduction into the worldwide juggernaut that is the "Vaccine Agenda".

There are now more than 200 vaccines and more coming - sounds good - but where have 1,000,000 autistic children come from, not to mention millions with HIV/AIDS? Why does a newborn baby need hepatitis B vaccine when hepatitis B comes from using dirty needles? Why does the medical industry not want a true anti-viral drug? These answers and more.

Just how many vaccines can our babies tolerate and what are the consequences of a few of the latest and greatest.

What is the real truth about AIDS - where did it come from and where is it going? There are so many unanswered questions - which is strange in itself. The death of Africa is unfolding before our eyes and there is money to be made for looking the other way. The unbelievable is both obvious and true. The true   origin of AIDS is revealed as well as the suppressed solution to the pandemic.

What have we learned? Well, if we have learned one thing, it's that the death toll is over 600,000 for useless drugs alone and countless millions more for failure to recognize really good drugs. Millions of hapless souls dutifully taking their prescribed pills-- secure in the certainty that they have not been misled. Can we ever recover from the debacle that is market and profit driven corporate control of modern medicine?   What are our real options and what remains of the so called "healthy lifestyle?"

"Discovery consists in seeing what everyone else has seen and thinking what no one else has thought"   Albert Szent - Gyorgi, 1937 Nobel Prize in medicine.

CHAPTER 1
VIOXX

In a lovely television commercial that most of us have seen, Dorothy Hamill is shown happily skating in circles, pain free, all due to the arthritis wonder drug for which pharmaceutical giant Merck spent over three hundred million dollars in direct advertising to the consumer. The Vioxx story has now laid bare the pattern of corruption and malfeasance which permeates the medical industry today.

Experts in testimony before a hearing of the Congress of the United States estimated that Vioxx caused one hundred sixty thousand unnecessary heart attacks and as many as sixty thousand deaths. Vioxx was approved by the FDA in May of 1999. In March of 2000, the VIGOR study disclosed that Vioxx had a 5 times greater cardiovascular risk than an alternate drug Naproxen. Between the time of the Vigor Study and withdrawal of Vioxx from the market September 30, 2004, Merck undertook a misleading promotional campaign to induce Doctor's to fill over one hundred million prescriptions resulting in more deaths than the Viet Nam War.

As a result of the many lawsuits instituted against Merck a huge array of documents and emails have surfaced-revealing the extent of Merck's malfeasance. These documents tell of Merck's systematic strategy to market a drug they knew to be dangerous, to mislead physicians and to conduct a policy of guest authored and ghost written medical studies. These studies were written by Merck employees and willing doctors were bribed to supply their names as guest authors in order to create suitable credibility. (See GUEST AUTHORSHIP AND GHOST WRITING IN PUBLICATIONS RELATED TO ROFECOXIB in JAMA April 16th, 2008- volume 299, no. 15.)

These revelations, unfortunately, are only the tip of the iceberg that threatens to destroy the scientific credibility of the entire pharmaceutical and medical publishing industries. Additionally, one must wonder where the FDA was during all this and also why did hundreds of thousands of doctors write millions of prescriptions for Vioxx after its safety was in question?

11

The sad truth is that Merck is not unique among drug companies in its methods of operation. Drug companies routinely bury studies showing that their drugs don't work.

A study recently published in the New England Journal of Medicine showed that more than one third of studies on antidepressant drugs go unpublished. Studies that were not positive and published were portrayed in a way that conveyed a positive outcome. The researchers examined 74 studies conducted on antidepressants between 1981 and 2004. Only 51% of these studies produced favorable results for the drugs being tested. All but one of those studies was published. In contrast 61% of the failed studies went unpublished. Of the 14 unfavorable studies published only 3 interpreted the data unfavorably. The other 11 studies cast the drugs as more effective as they actually were.

Of the 3 studies conducted on GlaxoSmithKline's Wellbutrin only the one showing positive was published. Of 5 studies conducted on Pfizer's Zoloft the one showing positive results was published, the one with questionable results was spun as if the drug was effective, and the 3 with unfavorable results were never published.

A study done by researchers at Johns Hopkins found that 100% of industry sponsored studies presented at an annual scientific meeting reported findings that support product use. (What a surprise!). To quote the authors, " With compelling evidence that the knowledge base produced by commercially sponsored research is biased, with evidence that physicians do not reliably detect bias in information presented to them, with no evidence that bias in individual studies is reliably detected and discounted, and with repeated examples of manufacturers using biased evidence to promote sales, what commercially supported research can be trusted? Drug companies corrupt science in a way that is directly harmful to patients."

So there we have it-- 100% is certainly astonishingly good luck--but where do we go from here? Certainly 110% should be attainable if we work at it. It is almost impossible to become an 'opinion leader' unless you do the clinical trials paid for by the pharmaceutical industry. These are the biggest, highest profile studies, and the results are presented at major medical meetings, and published in the high profile medical journals.

Ergo, opinion leaders are almost all supported and promoted by the industry. From the very start, they are a self-selected group; Pro-industry, pro-drug use. Usually, pro-specific drug.

These people write the editorials and speak to the press and take part in discussion and symposia and presentations. They are then invited onto prestigious committees that decide on the medical treatment for all of us.

Medical journals are no more than "an extension of the marketing arm of pharmaceutical companies" because a large proportion of their revenue comes from drug advertisements and reprints of company funded trials, claims former BMJ editor, Richard Smith.

Dr. Smith argues that although medical journals make a sizeable income from drug advertisements this is the least of their "corrupting form of dependence" on the industry, since the advertisements are "there for all to see and criticize."

Dr Smith's strongest criticism is leveled at the fact that journals publish clinical trials that are funded by the industry. Unlike advertisements, trials are seen by readers as the highest form of evidence, he says." Trials funded by drug companies rarely produce unfavorable results and make up between two thirds and three quarters of the trials published in key journals."

13

According to Dr. Malcolm Kendrick, an eminent critic of medical academia," some 'Opinion leaders' may be finding themselves a trifle uncomfortable with the stench of corruption. Nose plugs only work for so long. Here is a clip from an article found in a newsletter sent out to pharmaceutical executives.

Doctors Fight over Drug Firm Influence

A fierce, behind-the-scenes battle over how much influence drug companies exert on doctors is the raising blood pressure at the American Society of Hypertension.

The society's cofounder and long-time editor of the prestigious American Journal of Hypertension, Dr. John H. Laragh, has accused "academic physician/businessmen" who accept industry speaking and consulting fees of improperly colouring the group's activities.

"The lines separating marketing from education have been fractured," Laragh wrote in an e-mail message to physicians in the 3,000-member society.

The episode is a stark example of a broader debate taking place within the nation's medical societies, which represent physicians in virtually every medical specialty. Recently, many of the groups have become more sensitive to the potential for conflicts of interest relating to pharmaceutical industry grants.

Disagreements have flared over industry money used to support the hypertension society's educational programs, as well as the propriety of direct industry payments to physicians who serve as lecturers and consultants. The hypertension organization requires doctors participating in speaking programs to reveal the payments, but does not require them to disclose amounts.

Critics say the payments help companies put a patina of scientific and medical legitimacy on what is otherwise an attempt to increase market share.

"The society is seen as sort of a marketing tool by industry. There is a lot of money to go around," said Dr. Curt D. Furberg, a former member of its executive council and a professor of public health sciences at Wake Forest University in North Carolina.

Good for you Dr Furberg. You may not know who he is, but he has been making waves for years about the potential for calcium channel blockers (antihypertensives), to increase the overall mortality rate. This has made him particularly unpopular with those companies who make various calcium channel blockers. The word Pfizer springs to mind, for some reason.

It comes as no real surprise to see the academic world of hypertension research hitting the barriers first. Drugs to lower blood pressure were amongst the first to be subjected to massive marketing hype, and 'opinion leaders' in this area have had their snouts in the trough for longer than anyone else. Societies, such as the American Society of Hypertension are, basically, pharmaceutical company constructs.

To quote Dr Michael A. Weber (singled out for particular criticism by Dr Laragh).

All medical societies rely heavily on industry sponsorship, Weber said. "Otherwise we wouldn't exist,"

If the American Society of Hypertension wouldn't exist without industry sponsorship, then maybe it shouldn't exist at all."

Without going on, ad infinitum, it is seems clear that that the entire medical industry has failed to meet a fiduciary duty to protect the patients that they serve. This must include the pharmaceutical industry, the FDA, the medical journals, the entire research community, and last but not least the doctors who write the prescriptions. The doctors themselves remain the last gateway between deadly and ineffective drugs and a trusting patient population.

The reality is that none of us can exert even the smallest influence on this medical juggernaut that is nurtured and sustained by hundreds of billions of dollars generated by the promotion and sales of bad drugs. Therefore, we must attack this problem at its most vulnerable pressure point, that is, the doctors who are responsible for writing the prescriptions.

Drug companies are fond of telling people in their slick television commercials "ask your doctor if this drug is right for you" in their arrogant certainty that doctors are their sales lackeys and will do as they are told.

However, this is exactly what I am advising you to do, go to your doctor and ask if your drugs are right for you, but this time you will be armed with the information that will be available to you in the chapters following.

Following on the heals of the Vioxx debacle, Merck in it's overweening arrogance, joined with Schering Drug Company to sponsor a clinical trial called- ENHANCE- comparing the cholesterol lowering drug Vytorin, a combination of Zetia and Zocor, with Zocor alone. All of the data was analyzed by April 2006; however, not surprisingly, the results were not announced until January 14, 2008. This suppression allowed Merck and Schering to share in an additional ten billion dollars in revenue before the truth came out. Vytorin patients

16

developed more arterial plaque buildup than patients on Zocor alone, and Vytorin did not decrease the risk of heart attack or stroke. So much for learning their lesson from Vioxx!

The following chapters will go much deeper into the panorama of medical deception. As the reader progresses from one unbelievable scenario to the next the reader may be tempted to come to the conclusion that this is too much to believe, especially if it involves one of their own favorite drugs or medical modalities.

Please keep in mind that I am not providing you with my opinion, but I am drawing only on the data which the purveyors themselves have put forward.

The Journal of The American Medical Association (JAMA) has stated that prescription drugs in the normal course of use are the third leading cause of death in America. They estimate that over 106,000 die each year from prescription drugs, taken properly. I will prove in the following pages that not only do most of the drugs you are taking not work, **but the true number of deaths from commonly used medicines is over 700,000 per year, making legal drugs equal to cancer as a cause of death in America.**

The more we look into the pervasive patterns of deception utilized by all major drug companies the easier it will become to wean ourselves away from the delusion that they are our friends and can be trusted. U.S. Drug companies spend 2 times more money on marketing (50 billion dollars) than they do on research and development. **What they designate for research is primarily to promote their own brand of "me too" drug in the competition for market share.**

I have been searching diligently for a single drug developed by the pharmaceutical industry in the past fifty years that materially benefits any human disease. I am sure that many millions carrying little bottles of pills wherever they go truly believe that they are carrying their health and salvation with them. Sadly, nothing could be further from the truth. In the following chapters it will become clear, beyond any doubt, that the entire medical industry is complicit in perpetrating a massive fraud for money. Doctors themselves are the unwitting tools used by the pharmaceutical industry for this purpose.

Beyond this, the medical establishment has been so captured by their newfound celebrity and the windfall riches trickling down from the 700 billon dollar drug industry that they have closed ranks against any science or technology not in big pharma's failed agendas. The result of this is a death sentence for over 50 million people.

The elucidation of this pattern of malfeasance must be the first step in coming to grips with the truth. For we are embarking on a difficult journey in search of truth and there is no doubt that the reality that we are about to face will be incredibly difficult for most to accept. At first blush it will seem like a surreal fantasy concocted more from paranoia than objective observation. Nevertheless, as we progress from chapter to chapter and add piece after piece to the puzzle, somewhere along the way, despite our almost certain knowledge that it can't be true, the truth will strike. An undeniable, blinding reality. An epiphany of the obvious. An entire industry hoisted on the petard of their own making. **Their own clinical trial data** which they have obfuscated and misrepresented, hidden and buried, and just plain lied about. One by one the pillars which they have erected to support their version of reality will crumble and the unthinkable will be laid bare.

It is my hope that you will not find the data in the following pages onerous, as the devil is in the details, and the details are in the data. It is also my hope that what you read on the following pages will save your life.

CHAPTER II

IN THE BEGINNING

Not withstanding a few drug scandals are we not happier, healthier and living longer than every before? Certainly we are told that on a daily basis. Someone wants us to believe that very badly. So let us take a common sense look at the real results of our $2 trillion a year health care/pharmaceutical system.

Certainly the issues are complex and there are significant successes in medical care in America, but all is not well, so we will try to separate reality from mythology and wishful thinking.

The first and most prevalent certainty put forward as proof of success is what everyone knows --- that people are living longer than ever before.

It is often stated that the mean age of death today has increased to 77 as compared to 65 in 1960. But, what does this statistic really mean? It means that the mean or average age of death has shifted. Now this can happen in one of two ways. Either people are living longer or, as is the reality, fewer people are dying prematurely.

This decrease in early deaths is accounted for by a ten fold decrease in infant death rate, an almost 50% reduction in smoking, an almost 50% reduction in accidental deaths and a massive decrease in premature deaths from influenza and pneumonia. **The contribution of greater longevity to this shift is negligible.**

According to the US Census Bureau the percent of US population over age 60 in 1980 was 16.07%. In 2005--- it was 16.81%. Hardly a major march into the geriatric age!

Additionally, the progression to an older population is a global phenomenon unrelated to medical or pharmaceutical breakthroughs. For instance, in the same period which saw a 0.7% increase in the over 60 group in the United States, the over 60 group in Thailand increased by 4% and in Mexico increased by 2.5%.

20

According to the National Institute on aging in 1990 the 65-74 age group totaled 18 million. The 75 to 84 age group totaled 2 million and the 100 + age group was negligible. 15 years later in 2005 the 65 to 74 age group was 19 million. The 75 to 84 age group was 2 million and the over 100 age group remained negligible.

I think the point is clear that in all probability the "living longer" hypothesis is a myth.

A more meaningful statistic is the over all death rate per one hundred thousand persons. In 1960, the death rate in the US was 950 per thousand persons as compared to 820 today. A drop of less than 8% in half a century. Almost all of this reduction in death rate is accounted for by the same factors which led to the shift in the mean age of death discussed previously. In addition these numbers are biased by the so called "adjusted for age" data. If there is little true change in the crude figures their should be no need for a misleading age adjustment.

The three leading causes of death in the US are heart disease, cancer and stroke. Therefore much of the pharmaceutical/medical establishment deception is directed at these problems. Since the data is less complex we will take a look at cancer first.

Although there has been some progress in cancer salvage, particularly in childhood cancers, the overall cancer picture is dismal. If there ever was an egregious case of denial of failure, it is the cancer industry trumpeting victory over cancer death rates in 2004 called "turning the tide".

Cancer death rates decreased from 194 per one hundred thousand persons in 1950 to 186 deaths per one hundred thousand persons in 2004. **A decrease of a mere 4% in over half a century!** Without question, all of this decrease, and more, can be accounted for by a concomitant decrease in the rate of smoking of almost 50%. The CDC estimates that 30% of cancer deaths are directly related to smoking. They also estimate that cessation of smoking decreases the cancer risk by

50%. Therefore the reduction in smoking prevalence since 1950 should translate into a decrease in cancer deaths of at least 8%. So much for "Turning the tide!"

It is vital not to pass off rational and data- based criticism as a diatribe against scientific medicine. Proper science is the absolute key to incremental improvement in any discipline. However, passive acceptance of biased and erroneous science, created and interpreted by marketing and promotional entities, is far from the proper application of the scientific method.

We are facing now and in the near future an upswing of human disease of unprecedented proportions. There are massive increases in prevalence of cardiovascular disease, AIDS, SARS, bird flu, diabetes, Alzheimer's disease, arthritis and degenerative disease, autism, autoimmune disease and the list goes on.

We simply cannot afford to allow pharmaceutical mercenaries to dominate the medical machine leaving us a full half century behind in the technological explosion which has encompassed all other disciplines of science and human endeavor.

Chapter III
The Heart of the Matter

Cardiovascular disease is the leading cause of death in the US. Approximately 25% of the population suffers from some form of cardiovascular disease. Consequently, it is a major area of interest and profit for the pharmaceutical industry. Although a comprehensive analysis of all drugs relating to heart disease would more than fill this book on its own, I feel that we can get a close approximation of the actual state of affairs by concentrating on the key elements and the major prevalent misconceptions concerning heart disease in the 21 century .

As we look at clinical trial data it is important to bear in mind at all times that the inherent trustworthiness of these data is limited due by the liberal application of "tricks of the trade." The result is a clear bias exaggerating effectiveness and minimizing toxicity.

The New England Journal of Medicine refers to "publication bias" and estimates that failure to publish negative studies increases apparent drug effectiveness by 1/3. Other major factors resulting in overvaluations of a drug include; ghost writing, creating inclusion criteria allowing the selection of patients most likely to respond, using obviously ineffective double blinding techniques and simply stating the studies conclusions in as biased and positive a manner as possible.

Many of the studies are now written in a manner so complex that it forces the great majority of doctors to rely only on the simply stated proposition containing the key words "statistically significant effectiveness" and "well tolerated". In this way most doctors simply miss the fact that the data do not come close to justifying such a conclusion.

The most common and important technique to portray results as positively as possible is to report "relative risk reduction" instead of "absolution risk reduction". Relative risk reduction can appear quite large when absolute risk reduction is very small. If a disease kills two of every million people a drug that reduces the death rate to one in a million people would give a relative risk reduction of 50% which appears to be a benefit. **However, the absolute risk reduction is still only one in a million and one would have to treat one million people to achieve the saving of one life.** Moreover, the likely death rate from adverse events in the treated population would be catastrophic compared to the one life saved.

In-depth analyses of clinical trials indicate that drug tests sponsored by a pharmaceutical company show 90% positive results versus 50% positive results in independent non- drug sponsored studies. This factor is an additional bias unrelated to the process of burying negative studies discussed previously.

Confounding this scary situation is the fact that FDA approval of a drug is based only on a showing of "statistically significant" superiority over placebo (dummy pills) no matter how small the increment of superiority. This in no way is a measure of the true clinical efficacy of a drug or even the superiority of the drug over other drugs already in use.

The real meaning of "statistically significant" is that the numbers as shown are correct to a 95% probability-but this is totally unrelated to whether the drug has significant value. A drug showing effectiveness of 1% over placebo may be statistically significant, but will probably not be clinically significant, yet will achieve the all important FDA stamp of approval.

Another common practice is to test and present a drug for FDA approval based on a very minor and limited use. The drug company then markets the drug for "off label" use which magnifies its sale potential hugely without actually having to prove out its efficacy.

It is important to keep these factors in mind as we move now into the murky waters of cardiovascular therapy today. Above all, beware of studies that fail to mention or **show a decrease in overall death rate.** It would seem unlikely that most would willingly exchange a relatively easy death from a heart attack for a prolonged death from cancer.

In 2008 724,000 people died from cardiovascular disease and 147,000 people from stroke, making them the leading cause of death in America. The majority of drug therapies now used purporting to deal with cardiovascular disease have been instituted since 1990 and have continued to the present day.

A reduction in the heart disease death rate from 350 per one hundred thousand in 1960 to 260 per one hundred thousand today is universally attributed to these post 1990 drugs. It is worth noting, however, that the cardiovascular death rate from the period 1960 to 1990 fell at a rate of 6% per year whereas from 1990 to 2000, after the institution of these break-throughs, the rate of improvement fell to 2% per year, and from 2000 to 2002 it fell to .5% per year. Shouldn't this be the other way around?

Whatever the reason for this (does reduction in smoking come to mind?) the reduction in CVD death rate cannot be related to the institution of" better" drugs in the nineties.

As for the small gains seen in the last ten years they have almost certainly been due to improvement in surgical and angioplasty techniques as evidenced by a halving of the heart attack death rate in hospitals over the last decade which translates into more than 100,000 fewer deaths each year.

A lesser known but perhaps more telling statistic is that in 1960 heart disease accounted for 38% of deaths in the U.S.- Flashing forward to the year 2000 heart disease again accounted for 38% of deaths in the U.S. Apparently some statistics do not tell the whole story.

Four universally accepted modalities have been the cornerstones of the battle against heart disease since 1990. These include the cholesterol lowering **statin drugs,** (such as Lipitor), low dose **aspirin, low fat diet** and **antioxidants.** Is it possible that one or more, or perhaps all of these modalities are simply useless marketing ploys? Well, if you are to believe what I am about to divulge to you, it will be necessary to look into each one in depth so you can see the data and the truth with your own eyes. The judgment will be yours.

The properly medicated and informed person of today, at risk for a cardiovascular event, will be advised by his physician to be on a statin drug such as Lipitor, an aspirin daily (often with Plavix as well, a blood thinner), and to carefully maintain a low fat, low cholesterol diet.

Additionally he will be liberally ingesting dietary and supplemental antioxidants such as vitamin A, E, and C, which as everyone knows,(or think they know) protect you against aging and a host of other diseases, including heart disease and arthritis. He may or may not be exercising; since it is so much easier let the pills do the work.

If it has become clear that people are not actually living longer and are not healthier on this regimen, as we have suggested, it remains for us to examine each of these interventions in turn in order to elucidate the mystery.

Chapter IV

Beware of Cholesterol

The recent massive increase in the use of Lipitor, a statin drug, is based on a belief that there is major benefit to be derived from lowering serum cholesterol levels. The dictum that you can never get your cholesterol low enough has reached the level of religious dogma in the minds of every American. Prepare yourself for a major paradigm shift. It will become simply obvious from the most cursory viewing of the related data that this belief is totally false.

The first and most famous study regarding heart disease, diet and cholesterol levels was the Framingham Study started in the late 40's in Framingham, Massachusetts by the National Heart Institute. The objective of this study was to identify the common factors that contribute to cardiovascular disease and to follow its development over an extended period in a large number of participants. The project undertook to test the hypothesis that regulation of the level of serum cholesterol and the development of coronary heart disease are related to:

1. The caloric intake
2. The level of animal fat intake
3. The level of cholesterol intake

The results of the study were as follows:

1. The lower the caloric intake the higher the cholesterol level irrespective of physical activity.
2. No association was found between fat intake and cholesterol level, or between the ratio of plant fat to animal fat and cholesterol level.
3. No relationship was found between dietary cholesterol and serum cholesterol.

In a sixteen year follow-up no relationship was found between diet and subsequent development of cardiovascular disease.

Although the results were clear, Dr. William Kammell, the Director of the Framingham Study, obviously disappointed, made this remarkable statement "although there is no discernable relationship between diet intake and cholesterol levels in the Framingham Study group, it is incorrect to interpret this finding to mean that diet has no connection with serum cholesterol". This statement was a rather sinister; double speak clarification, ominously presaging the wave of hysteria to sweep the country as to the danger of high serum cholesterol.

It behooves us to examine more recent data that might refute or corroborate the results of the Framingham Study.

1965 a study published in the British Medical Journal divided heart patients into three groups. One group got corn oil, one group olive oil, and the third group was told to eat animal fat. **After two years the survival in groups one and two was 55%, however, the survival in the animal fat group was 75%.**

1966 a study published in the Journal of the American Medical Association compared two groups of New York business men. One group followed a so called "prudent diet" consisting of corn oil and margarine instead of butter, cereal instead of eggs, and chicken and fish instead of beef. A second group ate eggs for breakfast and meat three times a day. **The prudent dieters had average serum cholesterol of 220 compared with 250 in the eggs and meat group. At the end of the study there were 8 deaths from heart disease among the prudent diet group and 0 deaths among those who ate meat three times a day.**

1987 JAMA-Cholesterol and mortality, 30 year follow-up from Framingham Study. The study stated "there is a direct association between declining cholesterol levels and mortality." **There was found to be a 15% increased death rate for every 1 mmol/l drop in cholesterol level.**

30

1997 American Heart Association: effect of serum lipids on vascular and non vascular mortality in the elderly. "In a univariate analysis a **low total cholesterol level was associated with death due to both vascular and non vascular causes.** Neither concentration of HDL-C, LDL-C, triglycerides or apoB was associated with vascular or non vascular mortality. (That is, increased levels were associated with lower mortality!)

1998 Lancet- Total Cholesterol and the Risk of Mortality in the Oldest Old.
In seven hundred and twenty four participants over age 85 total cholesterol concentrations were measured and mortality risks calculated over ten years of follow-up.
Each one mmol/l increase in total cholesterol corresponded to a 15% decrease in mortality. Mortality from cancer and infection was significantly lower among the participants in the highest total cholesterol category.

2001 Lancet - Honolulu Heart Program.
Three thousand seven hundred and forty one men between 51 and 73 years of age were followed over 20 years to determine cholesterol levels relation to death rate. **The greatest death rate was found in those whose cholesterol levels were lowest** in both the 1971 and 1991 examinations. The earlier patients start to have lower cholesterol concentration the greater the risk of death. Death rate in the lowest cholesterol group was 69 per thousand as compared to 42 per thousand in the highest cholesterol group.

2006 A Tokai University Study surveyed 26 thousand people between 1987 and 2006.
Researchers found in terms of overall death men and women in the group with the **lowest LDL cholesterol-often called the bad cholesterol-had the highest death rate.**

31

The Multiple Risk Factor Intervention Trial; MRFIT:

This trial involved 361,662 high risk men in 28 medical centers at a cost of 115 million dollars. Their cholesterol intake was cut by 42%, saturated fat by 28% and total calories were cut by 21%. Coronary heart disease was unaffected. **The study's originators called the results "disappointing"** and said in their conclusions "The overall results do not show a beneficial effect on coronary heart disease or total mortality."

WHO European Coronary Prevention Study

The **results** of this study were **called "depressing"** because once again **no correlation between fats and heart disease** was found. There were more deaths in the lo-fat group than the control group.

A comprehensive meta-analysis of 26 studies published in 1992 concluded that "Lowering serum cholesterol concentrations does not reduce mortality and is unlikely to prevent coronary heart disease"

A Finnish trial in 1972 found in a 10 year follow-up, that **subjects who stayed on a cholesterol lowering diet were twice as likely to die of heart disease** as those who did not.

From the Journal of the American Family physician we find a study that examined whether the total cholesterol level would predict in-hospital mortality. The authors reviewed the hospital records at 81 different centers covering 6,984 study participants. **Pts with the lowest cholesterol levels had a mortality of 5.2%. Patients with the highest cholesterol** levels had a death rate of 1.6%. This is a **325% increased death rate with lower cholesterol.**

This inverse relationship holds in non-hospitalized deaths as well. A significant portion of these deaths should be attributed to the use of cholesterol lowering statin drugs such as Lipitor and Crestor--but they are not! Keep this number in mind when reading the following chapter on statins.

And to cap it all off, the largest ever cardiology study, which assessed 21 countries over 10 years-- The WHO-MONICA study--found no correlation between coronary heart disease and cholesterol levels. NONE..ZERO.. NO CORRELATION WHATSOEVER.

While we are on the subject The MONICA study proved beyond doubt that there is no correlation between saturated fat consumption and heart disease. The French consumed three times as much saturated fat as was consumed in Azerbaijan, and had one-eighth the rate of heart disease. Every single country in the top eight of saturated fat consumption had a lower rate of heart disease then every single country in the bottom eight of saturated fat consumption.

If you still believe that fat causes heart disease I give you the Woman's Health Initiative Heart Intervention study.

48,000 women were randomized and controlled. Half were put on lo-fat and high fruit, vegetable and grains diet. The study continued for 8 years. The results were as follows:

There was no significant difference in coronary heart disease or stroke incidence or mortality, or total mortality. The lo-fat diet also produced no reduction in cancer rates.

The response was predictable. Elizabeth Nabel M.D., director of the National Heart Institute had this to say." there may have been some "disappointment" that the studies didn't always give clear answers. The findings are what they are. Now we're in a second wave of putting the findings into perspective." [I translate this to mean "let's ignore these results and get on with it."]

Now let's get a few things straight. First: there is no relation between fat and cholesterol--none-- you cannot make cholesterol from fat. The only relation between the two is that both are carried around in lipo-proteins since neither is water soluble. The so called cholesterol blood levels are measures of lipo-protein not cholesterol (LDL and HDL).

Secondly, you cannot change LDL, HDL or "cholesterol" levels by eating or not eating fat or cholesterol and finally, neither fat intake nor cholesterol intake has anything to do with cholesterol levels and **cholesterol levels have nothing to do with heart disease.**

Research published in the European Journal of Nutrition found that 2 eggs daily added to a diet (British Heart Foundation) compared to those on the same diet but without eggs showed (surprise!) no change or reduction in cholesterol levels in both groups despite a fourfold increase in cholesterol intake in the egg eating group.

But this does not mean that cholesterol levels have nothing to do with mortality. In fact people with the lowest cholesterol levels have the highest mortality and people with normal or high cholesterol have the lowest mortality! Yes-- you are reading that correctly--if you missed it in the previous citations-- low cholesterol equals high mortality. Just in case you're still unconvinced-- let' take a quick look at more proof:

JOURNAL OF THE AMERICN GERIATRICS SOCIETY-- 2005 Plasma Lipids and all cause mortality in the Non-demented Elderly.
2277 participants age 67 to98.
Results: participants with levels of total cholesterol, HDL and LDL in the lowest quartile were twice as likely to die as those in the highest quartile. The risk of death was stronger for younger participants with low LDL (2.5 times).

JOURNAL OF AMERICAN CARDIOLOGY 2003 Gregg
Fonarow M.D., UCLA cardiomyopathy center.

"We first reported in 1998 that lower total cholesterol,
LDL, HDL and triglycerides were predictors of higher
mortality in 222 patients with heart failure with a risk ratio of
3.5. These results were surprising, counterintuitive and
received little attention.

We have recently reported on the relationship of
cholesterol, lipoproteins and mortality in 1134 patients with
heart failure of multiple etiologies. Low total cholesterol was a
strong, independent predictor of increased mortality. **Less
than 25% percent of patients in the lowest quartile
survived 5 years while survival was greater than 50% in
the two highest quartiles.**

In this issue of the Journal, Rauchaus et al report of two
cohorts of patients with chronic heart failure. In both cohorts
low levels of cholesterol were associated with higher mortality
rates. **The probability of survival increased by 25% for
each mmol/L increase in total cholesterol.** This was
independent of age.

The inverse relationship between mortality and lipid
levels has been observed in other disease states and
populations. Critical care literature provides strong evidence
for survival advantage associated with higher lipid levels.

Adverse outcomes associated with low serum cholesterol
have been reported in trauma, surgical illness, multiple organ
failure, dialysis and sepsis. Low serum cholesterol has also
been associated with worsened survival in the elderly".

Of course, it was advised that more clinical trials be done
before jumping to the conclusion that Statin therapy might be
associated with this increased death rate (no surprise there)

AMERICAN JOURNAL OF CARDIOLOGY 1981;
SERUM CHOLESTEROL AND MORTALITY   DJ.
KOZAREVIC

35

The relationship of serum cholesterol to all cause mortality over seven years in 11,121 males age 35-62 was determined. Those with lower cholesterol had a significantly higher mortality than those with higher cholesterol. This was significant and remained significant after adjusting for obesity, blood pressure, smoking, age and socio-economic status. Association between low cholesterol and deaths due to cancer and respiratory disease was significant.

A study in AMERICAN MEDICAL ASSOCIATION STROKE Journal reported that the risk of stoke in men of retirement doubled with low cholesterol (HDL).

A LANCET study in 1997 found that for every 1 mmol/L increase in cholesterol level in elderly patients there was a 15% decrease in overall mortality. Persons with high cholesterol levels were especially resistant to cancer and infections.

And saved for last, the study most despised and vilified by it's own researchers for daring to come up with unpalatable and "wrong" results unleashing a veritable litany of "pure speculation" as to the reasons that the study didn't come out the way it should have--we have THE HAWAIIAN HEART STUDY published in LANCET, Irwin Schatz M.D. professor of medicine at the University of Hawaii 2001.

3500 Japanese- American men over age 70 were studied. The death rate for those with lowest cholesterol was 68 per thousand per year while the death rate for those with the highest cholesterol levels was 43 per thousand per year. (Golly Gee! How could we have screwed this up so badly?)
Here's what Dr. Schatz had to say." we have been unable to explain our results. One proposed explanation is that this finding is somehow linked to this particular ethnic group" But then, giving a little more thought as to the absurdity of that

36

explanation he proceeds to say." We think it is reasonable to expand the conclusion to all Caucasian men".

But that really doesn't sound good either so he then goes on to give a possible explanation which he describes as "pure speculation" ---"I think a selection process takes place. People with high cholesterol below the age of 70 have increased mortality, and those that remain have been selected for survival."

Dr. Richard Stein, chief of cardiology at the Brooklyn Medical Center "speculates" on a different explanation. Low cholesterol levels could be an indication of an underlying medical problem.

Schatz says more research is needed to follow up the finding." Schatz adds." The central message is that we need a good, randomized trial of lipid lowering in the elderly. (Where have we heard that one before?)There is no need to change the basic recommendations that older people keep their cholesterol levels in check. "(What! But--what?) But he adds," I would suggest to physicians that they might want to be a little less aggressive in their efforts to lower cholesterol to very low levels in old people."(Didn't he just say that there was no need to change basic recommendations? Now I'm confused). And Dr. Stein says efforts to reduce heart disease by keeping cholesterol levels low should be pursued with" appropriate moderation" in older people.

And thus we simply substitute our learned opinions for all that sneaky and misleading data.

In the light of the preceding information it is more than difficult to understand how the entire medical establishment has accepted the cholesterol heart disease hypothesis with hardly a murmur of dissent. Nor is it understandable that they continue to deny their own data and continue to promote the "beware of cholesterol" fiction.

It is for this reason that I found it necessary to subject the poor reader to the preceding interminable litany of clinical studies showing all the same negative results. One could hardly believe the absolute and total contradiction that they portray to the recommendations of countless national and international advisory bodies, unless one was presented with the overwhelming body of evidence.

Contrary to everything one would hope for and imagine the vast majority of doctors appear to have fused into a monolithic and misled body, supported by arrogance, and fueled by pharmaceutical dollars. It would appear that the policy of providing physicians with huge amounts of sample drugs is a diabolical success. Just try to remember how pleased and grateful you were to your good doctor for giving you many free samples of an expensive drug. The doctor knows this, and the drug company knows that the doctor knows and the wheel is set in motion. What nobody cares to know is that most drugs kill many more than they save and the Doctor probably didn't even read the studies on the latest drug in their pretty sample packages that he just gave you.

Beyond all of this lies the greatest fear of all. If we give credence to our own data we will be forced to admit that that it is telling us that not only have we been 100% wrong, for all the wrong reasons, but that we are now solely responsible for hundreds of thousands of unnecessary deaths! That's pretty strong motivation to fail to be able to explain the results of our own studies.

This failed system in its overweening arrogance set the stage for the ushering in of the greatest corporate bonanza in history-- Lipitor.

Chapter V

Enter Lipitor

Statin drugs crept onto the market to save us from the disease of "high serum cholesterol", a disease without signs or symptoms. A disease where people actually feel good and can only be detected by the doctor's blood test.

Statin drugs block the enzyme that is necessary for the production of cholesterol. They do this very well, but unfortunately, they also block production of a vital cellular nutrient, co-enzyme Q10. Side effects of Q10 deficiency include muscle wasting; heart failure, neuropathy and cell membrane leakage. Cholesterol is vital to proper neurological function and is a precursor to all hormones produced in the adrenal gland.

Thus the disruption of cholesterol production can be expected to have a broad spectrum of serious and even catastrophic side effects.

Lipitor, the most popular statin drug, entered the market as a miracle cure for the "disease" of high or even normal serum cholesterol with the promise of a breakthrough in the control of cardiovascular disease. The media blitz and promotional efforts were unprecedented. They enlisted advertising agencies, scientific associations, heart disease foundations, doctors, researchers and anyone else they could buy. Sixteen million Americans now take Lipitor at a cost of twenty billion dollars a year. Just what are we getting for our money?

The answer to this question resides in a careful analysis of the results of many clinical trials. Apparently the way in which the doctors do it, is to fish around among these trials until they find one that tells them what they want to hear and is, preferably, sponsored or written by a major drug company. Often, finding that study itself is presented in a rather long and complex manner, they skip to the conclusion and read the magic words "effective and well tolerated"-- always quick and easy to understand. They then wait for one of the drug companies thousands of detail men (drug representatives) to fill them in on the rest of what they need to know. Doctors, in general, don't seem to know what we now know--that drug company studies have to be viewed with a high suspicion of bias and that "statistically significant" does not mean clinically significant.

It is interesting and unfortunate that studies that fail to show efficacy are often attacked and criticized whereas studies that purport to show efficacy are rarely criticized. The studies that are criticized and ignored are often independent studies with negative findings.

Studies with negative findings always are couched with the word "may" as, for example, a study finding that there is a much higher incidence of hemorrhagic stroke in older persons will headline "Aspirin **may** increase risk of stroke in the elderly" alternately, if a study finds a decrease in the incidence of stroke the headline will say" Aspirin **reduces** the risk of stroke in women 17%". This simple technique serves to make light of an important negative finding and over-values an insignificant positive finding.

The slight of hand is everywhere one looks. Almost universally, when a study fails to corroborate entrenched thinking, the researchers become abjectly apologetic and proffer reasons why the data might be flawed----actually criticizing their own study design and suggesting that further studies might provide a different(more acceptable) result.

On the other hand studies which find "statistically significant" results that are in the direction that the researchers want or prefer are never criticized or second guessed. I have yet to read a clinical trial that questions whether a finding of a reduced risk of one tenth of a percent a year compared to placebo might not be of clinical significance. Rarely have I read the suggestion that the likelihood of adverse events or side effects renders such a marginal benefit unacceptable.

In the previous chapter on cholesterol we have seen why it is so vital that data showing a mortality benefit for higher cholesterol levels simply cannot be accepted. This issue is inextricably intertwined with the lavish praise heaped upon statin drugs due to the love affair between Medicine and the pharmaceutical industry. If the data were to be accepted as

41

true, doctors must face the reality that they have been hoodwinked into killing hundreds of thousands of patients by the aggressive use of statin drugs. So here is the preposterous result of their pompous denial of their own data----

Several studies demonstrated a much greater death rate in dialysis patients with low cholesterol than in patients with high cholesterol. Obviously this could not be allowed to stand. Researchers at Johns Hopkins immediately published a study (Johns Hopkins and the pharmaceutical industry seem to have more than excellent relations) purporting to show that this "anomaly" could "likely" be explained by the cholesterol lowering effects of inflammation and malnutrition common in dialysis patients. They then proceeded to show signs of these problems in a cohort of patients with a battery of lab tests. **Although overall lower cholesterol levels were associated with higher mortality, we should not let that confuse us says Dr.Yongmei Liu M.D.,** He says, "The same serum cholesterol means different things depending on the presence or absence of inflammation". Just to add emphasis to this rather murky and unconvincing repudiation of the observed data, Dr.Jacques Rossouw of the National Institute of Health (NIH) had this to say, "Data linking low cholesterol with excess mortality have been gathered from both observational and clinical trials. Likely explanations of the association are that low cholesterol is a consequence of disease or is a confounder associated with other variables. (It seems never to occur to them that early studies showing high cholesterol to be a risk factor in men under 50 were a consequence of being a confounder associated with other variables!)

The authors conclude that evidence "suggesting" low cholesterol as a cause of excess mortality currently lacks breadth and rigor, and find no basis for changing cholesterol management guidelines."(Dare I point out here that the majority of the studies, then and now, explicitly state that their results were independent of the presence of inflammation or malnutrition.)

So what can remain of the evidence so lacking in breadth or vigor? Well, just for starters:

STROKE 2007 AMERICAN HEART ASSOC.: Post stroke mortality was inversely related to cholesterol level. Stroke severity was also inversely related to cholesterol level. The lower the cholesterol level the more severe the stroke.

JOURNAL OF AMERICAN GERIATRICS 2005 RELATIONSHIP BETWEEN PLASMA LIPIDS AND ALL CAUSE MORTALITY IN THE NON DEMENTED ELDERLY: 2,277 PARTICIPANTS age 65 to 98:
Participants in the lowest quartile of cholesterol level were twice as likely to die as were those with the highest cholesterol levels. This correlation was strongest in the youngest participants who had 2.5 times the death rate.

EUROPEAN HEART JOURNAL 1997:
A study on 11,500 patients over 3 years showed 2.2 times increased risk of death in low cholesterol group. Primarily due to increased risk of cancer.

JAMA 1987:
"There is a direct association between falling cholesterol levels over the first 14 years (of the Framingham study) and mortality over the following 18 years. 11% overall and 14% CVD death rate increase per 1mg/dl per year drop in cholesterol levels.

JOURNAL OF CARDIAC FAILURE 2002:
Tamara and associates report on their analysis of 1134 patients with heart disease that low cholesterol was associated with worse outcomes and impaired survival. Elevated cholesterol was not associated with hypertension, diabetes, or coronary heart disease.

43

AMERICAN HEART JOURNAL 2008:

17,791 Patients with congestive heart failure were analyzed according to cholesterol level .those in the highest quartile had the lowest risk of death 1.3%. Those in the lowest quartile had the highest risk of death 3.3%. For each 10mg. increase in cholesterol level mortality was decreased by 4%.

AMERICAN FAMILY PHYSICIAN 2005:

4309 patients age 65 years and older were followed over 3 years. The death rate in low cholesterol patients was twice those in high cholesterol range. These findings were independent of factors which might be indicative of nutritional or physical decline.

EUROPEAN HEALTH MONITORING PROGRAM 2004:

149,000 participants age 20 to 95 years followed for 15 years. The researchers observed that low cholesterol was significantly associated with increased all cause mortality in men across the entire age range, and in women from the age of 50 onward. Low cholesterol showed significant associations with death from cancer, liver diseases, and mental diseases. The researchers remarked that "the low cholesterol effect occurs even among younger respondents, contradicting the previous assessments, among cohorts of older people, that this is a marker for frailty occurring with age."

THE GERONTOLOGICAL SOCIETY OF AMERICA 2004:

Mortality of older patients with ischemic stroke. Mortality was 2.17 times higher in patients with low versus normal or high cholesterol.

THE MULTIPLE RISK FACTOR INTERVENTION TRIAL:

The authors examined the relation between serum cholesterol level and the risk of death in 350,977 men aged 35-57. The study found the risk of death from stroke was three times higher in men with low serum cholesterol levels.

So are we to believe the drug companies and their spokespersons at the NIH and Johns Hopkins, or our own lying eyes? If they are right and the "cholesterol causes heart disease" hypothesis is correct, than their statin drugs should not only be hugely lifesaving but should show a linear benefit with cholesterol lowering--but do they?

We will again look at what they look at and let's see if we see what they see. Doctors do an excellent job of convincing their patients, as they write a prescription, that if they don't take this pill they are balancing on the knife edge of a massive heart attack or other catastrophe - disconcerting indeed --- but, not to worry, Lipitor changes all that. Well, let's see if you agree:

"OVER -VIEW OF STATIN STUDIES 1992 - 2000". The results of all major studies up to the year 2000:

THE FOUR S, WOSCOPS, CARE, AFCAPS and LIPID STUDIES - generally showed only small, often statistically insignificant, differences independent of cholesterol lowering effect. In two studies mortality was higher in the statin treated group and **in no study was overall mortality lower in the treatment group compared to placebo.**

A meta-analysis of twenty six controlled studies found an equal number of cardiovascular deaths in the treatment and controlled groups in **a greater number of total deaths in the treatment groups.** Analysis of all large trials prior to 2000 for primary prevention of heart disease showed a **1% greater** mortality of treated subjects over a 10 year period compared to placebo.

Do more recent studies show a different result? We shall see.

45

MIRACL "2001"

High dose Lipitor was tested on 3086 in hospital for myocardial infarction or angina (chest pain). **No change in death rate compared to placebo.**

PROSPER
Pravastatin versus placebo. Pravastatin did not reduce total M.I. or stroke in the primary prevention population --or show any difference in total mortality.

ALLHAT (2002)
The largest North American cholesterol lowering trial ever, using Lipitor, showed **equal mortality in the treatment group and controls.** (10,365 participants). There was a non-significant decrease in total cardiovascular events.

METASTUDY ANALYSIS (2003)
An analysis of 44 trials totaling ten thousand patients showed **death rates on statins and placebo to be equal.** 65% of people on statin treatment suffered adverse events.

STATINS AND PLAQUE (2003)
Researchers examined coronary plaque buildup in 182 subjects divided into high dose and low dose statins. Using electronic beam tomography patients were studied for one year. Both groups showed an increase in plaque buildup of 9.2%.

STATIN AND WOMEN (2003)
No study has shows a reduction in mortality in women treated with statin. The University of British Columbia therapeutic initiative stated that statins offered no benefit to women for prevention of heart disease.

ASCOTT -LLA (2003)

Ten thousand participants (This is the study doctors really like to quote - let's see if you find it as compelling). This study showed a 1% decrease in non fatal heart attacks in men over a period of 3.5 years, this is equal to 0.28% per year. There was a 0.5% decrease in fatal MI and non fatal strokes over a period of 3 years. This equals a 0.14% decrease per year compared to placebo.

There was no difference in all cause mortality between the treated and placebo groups.

According to this data it would be necessary to treat 350 people, without benefit, for one year, to prevent 1 non fatal MI. In addition it would be necessary to treat 700 persons, without benefit, for 1 year to prevent 1 non fatal stroke.

According to Dr. Norton M. Hadler, Professor of Medicine, at the University of North Carolina "anything over an NNT (number needed to treat) of 50 is worse than a lottery". Several recent scientific papers pegged the NNT for statins at 250 and up even if they take it for 5 years or more.

Here is the heralded "breakthrough" study purported to confirm the efficacy of statins:

PROVE-IT (2004) versus J-LIT (2002)

The prove- it study led by research at the Harvard University Medical School attracted immense media attention. This is the study Pfizer ballyhoos in their TV ads. A New York Times headline stated "study of 2 cholesterol drugs finds 1 halts heart disease". The Washington Post chimed in with "striking benefits found in ultra low cholesterol". -- So much for being able to believe in a newspaper headline. I am sure that virtually no one knew how incredibly absurd these headlines were when they read them, or even know to the present day. This media blitz was the opening salvo in the battle to open the door to giving statins to normal, low risk,

47

healthy people - what a windfall to Pfizer - looking to put everybody who walks upright on Lipitor!

I suspect that no study in the history of medicine (with one exception) is more demonstrative of the propensity of the medical establishment to delude, mislead and deceive their unsuspecting patients - and perhaps even themselves. The reader will have to pay careful attention to the following exposition so as not to miss the "slight of hand" that manages to portray something positive out of absolutely nothing.

PROVE-IT divided 4162 patients into two groups. One group received Lipitor and second group another statin drug, Pravachol. The Lipitor group had a greater reduction in LDL cholesterol (95 versus 62 for Pravachol). The study then claimed a 16% greater reduction in all cause mortality for the Lipitor group.

The conclusion one is supposed to draw is that, the more one lowers the cholesterol, the more one lowers the death rate. Unfortunately, this slight of hand is easy to see through. Firstly, a 16% mortality rate represents a relative risk reduction. The absolute death rate for those on Lipitor was 2.2% and on Pravachol 3.2% over a period of two years, a difference of 0.5% per year. This difference although certainly small, is not nearly as important as that we are supposed to ignore the fact that-- the two groups were each on an entirely different drug--- which means that any difference, however, small must be related to the difference in the drugs used rather than any difference in cholesterol levels between the groups!

A final point to be made is that a better, larger, longer study done two years earlier - the J-LIT Study - with ten times the patient population (47,294)over 6 years resulted in no correlation between he amount of LDL lowering and death rate and HDL levels showed an inverse relationship with coronary events. This was a far more definitive study which, not surprisingly, was ignored by the media. This also shows that there is an obvious pattern of preferential cherry picking of studies more acceptable to the medical community.

THE SPARCL STUDY (2006) High dose Atorvastatin after stroke or ischemic attack
    4,730 patients were assigned to 80mg Lipitor or to placebo. The primary end point was to be a first stroke. The follow up was 4.9 years. The Lipitor group had a total of 273 strokes while the placebo group had a total of 307 strokes. Hemorrhagic stroke in the Lipitor group was higher than in the Placebo group (55 versus 33). The absolute decrease in the Lipitor group was 0.4% per year. **In overall mortality there were 5 more deaths in the Lipitor group compared with the placebo group.**
    Lipitor had a greater death rate or mortality than placebo and to prevent 1 non fatal stroke per year it is necessary to treat 500 patients who receive no benefit, but all the side effects.
    On the basis of this data the New England Journal of Medicine published in its conclusion the following: "80mg daily of Atorvastatin reduced the overall incidence of stoke, despite a small increase in the incidence of hemorrhagic stroke". They did not see fit to mention that the death rate from hemorrhagic stroke is 80% compared to a death rate of 10% for ischemic stroke. It has also been shown that the death rate for ischemic stoke is three times higher in men with low serum cholesterol levels! (Multiple Risk Factor Intervention Trial)
    For the final "nail in the coffin" (no pun intended), I refer you to the ignominious end of Pfizer's much hoped for miracle drug Torcetrabib. Scientists had seen Torcetrabib as the vanguard of a new wave of medicine that would give physicians new ways to reduce heart disease by raising "good cholesterol".
    Three years and hundreds of millions of dollars into the ILUMINATE study of Torcetrabib; the trial was summarily canceled when 82 people on the drug died as compared to 51

49

in the control group. Similar discrepancies were seen in all other cardiovascular problems. Again we see increased mortality with a statin.

As I write this chapter Astra Zeneca has released the results of yet another study on Crestor in 2008--proclaiming almost 50% reduction in total cardiovascular events and ever broadening the category of people that they claim should be on this drug. Despite the litany of contrary data that we have now seen, it is apparent I must address one more study now being trumpeted as a major breakthrough by an adoring media and a hoodwinked medical establishment.

At this point, you may be asking yourself why I think I am so much smarter than most other doctors in the world. The truth is I'm as perplexed about that as you are. I have, from time to time, tried to make sense of that concern in this book.

They certainly have the same access to the data that I have and their interpretation always seems far more favorable. They just seem to be caught in the mental gymnastic that says "it must be good if everyone is saying that it's good". In any event, we certainly can use our own brains to decipher the data without being caught in that trap.

As far as the "latest" Crestor study is concerned (JUPITER), the first thing to be aware of is that all subjects were among people with a high" C-reactive protein" lab value, indicative of a non-specific inflammatory process. Therefore, this study is not applicable to the general population even if the results were meaningful---which they are not.

Since it appears that high cholesterol no longer seems to qualify as a" disease ", perhaps they can succeed in convincing us that a high" C-reactive protein" lab value is a" disease "that we should treat with their drug. After all they have convinced us that a high Cholesterol lab result was a"disease"for many years. Just what does their" new disease" study data really say?

In 10,000 subjects for one year there were 30 less cardiac" events" in the treated group or a reduction of approximately .03 %. This is not 3% but three tenths of one per cent. No study can claim that level of precision, much less one done by a drug company and following dozens of other failed studies.

Even if we accept the data as meaningful and agree that 30 events per year were avoided (or more likely delayed) and if we assume the mortality of these 30 to be 3% (Usual in hospitalized elderly) we would have saved 1.0 life by treating 10,000 persons at a cost of $12 million. Or would we?

Dr. Wolfe of "Public Citizen" in a letter published in the journal Lancet reported that the rate of kidney damage in Crestor patients is 75 times higher than in patients taking other statin drugs. By 2004 there had been 29 reports of kidney failure. Also by 2004 there were 65 reports of rhabdomyolosis among U.S. patients taking Crestor making it as dangerous as Baycol, a statin drug which was withdrawn from the market in 2001.

Health Canada and the U.S. FDA have advised that patients be given the lowest possible dose of Crestor because of the associated adverse side effects. Keep in mind that serious adverse effects would most certainly increase with longer use and not necessarily be seen within the short time frame of clinical trials.

Finally, the long term increased mortality we have seen in patients with lower cholesterol due to Crestor(and other statins) would dwarf any purported positive benefit and these deaths would not be attributed to Crestor(15% increase in mortality for every point decrease in cholesterol level). In the 17 million now on Crestor this would translate into more than 150,000 deaths per year or in the clinical trial cohort of 10,000, where Crestor prevented 1.0 death, there would be 88 deaths at a later time!

Now I invite you, do you agree with my concerns or with the adoring praise of the medical establishment? If you agree with me, you have your answer-- if not the reason why.

The following quotes are the response to this clinical trial (JUPITER) which demonstrated no mortality benefit whatsoever with Crestor:

"A highly anticipated study has produced powerful evidence that a simple blood test can spot seemingly healthy people who are at increased risk for a heart attack or stroke and that giving them a widely used drug offers potent protection against the nation's leading killers." -Rob Stein, the Washington Post

"The potential public health benefits are huge. It really changes the way we have to think about prevention of heart attack and stroke." - Paul M. Ridker of the Brigham and Women's Hospital in Boston.

"It's a breakthrough study, it's a blockbuster. It's absolutely paradigm-shifting." - Steven E. Nissen of the Cleveland Clinic. (These are the words drug companies want to hear.)

"This takes prevention to a whole new level. Yesterday you would not have used a statin for a patient whose cholesterol was normal. Today you will." - W. Douglas Weaver, president of the American College of Cardiology.

"These are findings that are really going to impact the practice of cardiology in the country." -Dr. Elizabeth G. Nabel, director of the National Heart, Lung and Blood Institute.

It should now be strikingly apparent that there is a total disconnect between the data and the incomprehensible and delusional response of the medical community to a study which the most casual observers would label as a total failure. No-one seems to have noticed that this study was only on people with so called "normal cholesterol levels" which totally

52

repudiates the preposterous dogma that statins provide benefit by lowering cholesterol levels! They have abandoned their own hypothetical rationale driving the use of statin drugs for twenty years in the blink (or wink) of an eye.

I can hardly end this chapter without mention of one final" proof" of the value of statin drugs if only to demonstrate the failure of researchers to understand the implications of their own research.

The Veterans Administration followed almost one million veterans comparing death curves between those on statin drugs and those not on statin drugs. The data demonstrated a mean age of death 1.8 years longer for the statin group. Their conclusion was that statins demonstrate a longevity benefit. Unfortunately no-one seemed to want to recognize the true import of the study--the essential difference between the two groups was cholesterol level, since those on statins were high and those not on statins were low and it has been clearly shown that higher cholesterol confers a survival benefit.

The effect of statin use was to truncate and reduce the survival benefit of higher cholesterol, as evidenced by the fact that the tail of the survival curve was absent in the statin group--i.e. far fewer in the statin group lived beyond 90 as compared to the non- statin group. For the study to be meaningful, the two cohorts must be randomized and equal at baseline, with equal cholesterol levels. What they really accomplished was to reduce the longevity benefit of higher cholesterol. [How do you think they could have missed that point?]

This brings us directly to a subject that has been, in general, missing from the previous discussion, and that is, what do 500 people taking these drugs, without benefit, have to pay in adverse events and side effects for the Possible benefit to one.

CHAPTER VI
A PRICE TO PAY

Doctors have a propensity for ignoring side effects and adverse reactions from the drugs they give to their patients. It has been estimated that less than 5% of adverse drug reactions are reported. When the true efficacy of a drug is miniscule or non existent, even a small percentage of adverse events destroys any pretense of a positive "risk - benefit ratio" that the doctors are so fond of postulating. Obviously small benefits are quickly obliterated by even small numbers of serious adverse events. This is the final and total unraveling of any rational argument for the use of statin drugs.

Pfizer lists the following reported adverse events for Lipitor at 2% or less frequency in clinical trials (Please excuse me for putting this lengthy document in- but it's got to be seen).

Body as a whole: Chest pain, face edema, fever, neck rigidity, malaise, photosensitivity reaction, generalized edema.

Digestive system: nausea, gastroenteritis, liver function abnormality, colitis, vomiting, gastritis, dry mouth, rectal hemorrhage, esophagitis, eructation, glossitis, mouth ulcerations, anorexia, increase appetite, stomatitis, biliary pain, cheilitis, duodenal ulcer, dysphagia, enteritis, melena, gum hemorrhage, stomach ulcer, tenesmus, ulcerative stomatitis, hepatitis, pancreatitis, cholestatic jaundice.

Respiratory system: bronchitis, rhinitis, pneumonia, dyspnea, asthma, epistaxis.

Nervous system: insomnia, dizziness, paresthesia, somnolence, amnesia, abnormal dreams, decreased libido, emotional liability, in-coordination, peripheral neuropathy, torticollis, facial paralysis, hyperkinesias, depression, hypesthesia, hypertonia.

Musculoskeletal: arthritis, leg cramps, bursitis, tenosynovitis, myasthenia, tendinous, contracture, myositis.

Skin and appendages: Pruritus, contact dermatitis, alopecia, dry skin, sweating, acne, urticaria, eczema, seborrhea, skin ulcer.

Urogenital system: urinary tract infection, hematuria, albuminuria, urinary frequency, cystitis, impotence, dysuria, kidney calculus, nocturia, epididymitis, fibrocystic breasts, vaginal hemorrhage, breast enlargement, metrorrhagia, nephritis, urinary incontinence, urinary retention, urinary urgency, abnormal ejaculation, uterine hemorrhage.

Special senses: amblyopia, tinnitus, dry eyes, refraction disorder, eye hemorrhage, deafness, glaucoma, parosmia, taste loss, taste perversion.

Cardio vascular system: palpitation, vasodilatation, syncope, migraine, postural hypotension, phlebitis, arrhythmia, hypertension.

Metabolic and nutritional disorders: peripheral edema, hyperglycemia, creatine phosphokinase increase, gout, weight gain, hypoglycemia.

Hemic lymphatic system: ecchymosis, anemia, lymphadenopathy, thrombocytopenia, petechia.

Adverse events associated with Lipitor therapy reported after market introduction, which are not listed above, include the following: anaphylaxis, angioneurotic edema, erythema multiforme, Stevens - Johnson syndrome, toxic epidermal necrolysis, rhabdomyolysis leading to kidney failure, fatigue, tendon rupture.

The only missing side effect from Lipitor would appear to be loss of sense of humor. Of course, some of the side effects maybe unrelated to Lipitor and may be incidental, but one would have to be Bozo the clown or a Pfizer employee to believe that Lipitor was not responsible for a significant portion of these adverse events.

Let us examine what other sources tell us about Lipitor. Dr. Beatrice Golomb headed a study at the University of California San Diego assessing statin side effects. The industry insists that only 2 to 3% of patients get muscle pain and cramps, but Golomb found that over 90% of patients taking Lipitor and 1/3 of patients taking Mevacor (lower dose) suffered from muscle problems. The FDA withdrew Bayer's statin drug Baycol from the market due to a high incidence of life threatening cases of rhabdomyolosis.

According to the UCSD Study, nerve problems are a common side effect. Patients on statins for 2 or more years are at 4 to 14 fold increased risk of polyneuropathy. Dr. Golomb reports that in many cases patients told her that they had complained to their doctors about neurological problems only to be assured that their symptoms could not be related to cholesterol lowering medications. The damage from polyneuropathy is often irreversible.

Deaths attributed to heart failure have more than doubled from 1989 to 1999 - statin drugs were approved for use in 1989.

Cardiologist Peter Langsjoen studied 20 patients with normal heart function. After 6 months on Lipitor 2/3 showed significant abnormalities in the heart's filling phase. Not withstanding, virtually all patients with heart failure are put on statin drugs.

Researchers in the UK followed 114 heart failure patients. Survival was 78% at 12 months and 56% at 36 months. **They found that for every point decrease in serum cholesterol there was a 36% increase in risk of death within 3 years.**

Fifteen percent of statin patients develop some cognitive side effects. The most harrowing involve global transient amnesia - complete memory loss for a brief or lengthy period. In a trial involving 2500 subjects, amnesia occurred in 7 receiving Lipitor.

Many studies in animals show that statins cause cancer. In the heart protection study skin cancer occurred in 243 patients treated with Simvastatin compared with 200 patients in the control group.

An extensive over- view of efficacy and safety of statin was conducted and published by the Presidential Medical Center of Moscow, which stated the following:

In the majority of randomized controlled trials of therapy with statin, the results of which were analyzed separately for men and women, no lowering of rates of coronary events were found among women and people older than 65 years. More over, in some trials increases of all cause mortality were observed in statin treated patients at the account of deaths from non-cardiovascular causes (cancer deaths in particular).

In the PROSPER trial Prevastatin not only turned out useless in men and women over age 70, but significantly increased rates of breast cancer

. In ALLHAT-LLT in patients age 65 years and older and in women Prevastatin lowered neither total numbers of non- fatal myocardial infarctions and ischemic heart disease deaths, nor total mortality.

In SPARCL and TNT in which the efficacy and safety of high dose statin (that is Atorvastatin 80mg-day) was accessed there occurred augmentation of hemorrhagic stroke and mortality from non cardiovascular causes including cancer and infections.

One of the meta-analyses revealed a significant increase in breast cancer risk associated with treatment with statin. In another meta-analysis close relationship was noted with the development of cancer in elderly patients.

Lastly, I would encourage anyone who prescribes, takes or is thinking about taking a statin drug to Google ALS(Lou Gehrig's disease) and Lipitor and read what the many unfortunate
victims are trying to tell us:
(http://www.communicationagents.com
/sepp/2006/10/07/Lipitor_neurological_side_effect
_amyotrophic_lateral_sclerosis_alzheimers.htm).

Beyond this, the monetary cost of a useless treatment is astronomical -- exceeding twenty billion dollars a year. An honest assessment of the foregoing information should make it impossible to conclude that there is any legitimate use for a statin drug.

I will quote Texas cardiologist Dr. Peter Langsjoen, who said it best, "statin drugs are appropriate only as a treatment for cases of advanced cholesterol neurosis, created by the industries' anti- cholesterol propaganda. If you are concerned about your cholesterol a statin drug will relieve you of your worries".

CHAPTER VII
AN ASPIRIN A DAY

Fifty million Americans take an aspirin daily, hoping to ward off a fatal or debilitating heart attack or stroke. Aspirin use is arbitrarily divided into two categories, "primary prevention," that is, prior to a heart attack or stroke and "secondary prevention" after a heart attack or stroke. The second category contains different types of acute situations such as acute MI.

For all intents and purposes clinical trials data applies equally to treatment in both groups with the exception of acute situations. It is not within the scope of this book to analyze the data on all conditions that may be considered acute, except to state the following:

In all of these sub groups, that are at extreme high risk and need to be treated with a blood thinning agent, it would be most appropriate to utilize Warfarin (coumadin). I will refer you to an article in:

"Cardiology Review" entitled "Warfarin versus aspirin for stroke prevention in the elderly":

Twenty seven clinical trials have demonstrated the over whelming advantage of Warfarin to aspirin therapy on prevention of atrial fibrillation related stroke - reporting an efficacy of 60% compared with 20% with aspirin. The BAFTA Study showed conclusive and striking results. Patients followed for 2.7 years suffered 3.8% stroke on aspirin compared to 1.8% of patients on Warfarin. Further more, this benefit was not offset by hemorrhagic complications in the Warfarin group and even the incidence of extra cranial hemorrhage was lower in the Warfarin than in the aspirin group - 1.4% versus 1.7%. **This data should be applicable to all acute and high risk patients.**

Returning to the clinical trials applicable to the 50 million low and high risk subjects popping an aspirin daily, I might as well let the cat out of the bag immediately. Aspirin for this multitude of persons for prevention of heart attack and stroke is totally without merit, and in all probability, is a cause of increased morbidity and mortality.

As you have now seen the previous data on statin drugs, you may now be willing to give this remarkable statement some credence. It will become clear that not one life has been saved, and aspirin is no more a shield against heart attack and stroke than is Lipitor.

As with Lipitor the perpetration of the aspirin dogma requires the willing participation of the same categories of sacrosanct and prestigious medical experts that have given us Lipitor and the cholesterol hoax - now we have; "pop an aspirin a day and keep heart attack away".

One has to wonder how all the people involved in such a massive deception remain totally sanguine during their endless pontification and discussion of data that even the most unsophisticated lay person would label as garbage- If I am putting this in excessively strong terms it is only due to the fact that the deception is so egregious as to be totally inexcusable.

So, as we did with the statin drug, lets look at the real story about aspirin, "the miracle drug", and cardiovascular disease. Try not to miss the "slight of hand" that almost qualifies the medical magicians for prosecution under the RICO act. I must apologize for the following litany of studies---- but I cannot just leave you with only my opinion---you just would not believe me.

From CARDIOVASCULAR MEDICINE - Stanford University- we learn the following:
"In the SAPAT TRIAL of 2500 men with angina pectoris, the study failed to demonstrate an all cause mortality benefit.

Similarly, the PHYSICIANS HEALTH STUDY failed to demonstrate a mortality benefit. Two other studies PARS and AMIS failed to demonstrate a mortality benefit."

Amazingly, on the basis of these studies the ACCP recommendation is that patients with chronic coronary disease take 160mg to 355mg aspirin per day.

At this point one might wonder what would be the impetus to continue financing failed clinical trials, ad infinitum. The answer is that these trials serve the purpose not of true research, but as sales promotional tools, as well as a way to pass huge funds into the medical community who's "loyalty" they wish to buy.

Continuing with the litany of "impressive" randomized and controlled clinical trials we have:

BRITISH DOCTORS TRIAL - BDT 5139 patients studied over 5.8 years - no significant difference was demonstrated between aspirin and placebo in non fatal MI, non fatal stroke or cardiovascular mortality.

PHYSICIANS HEALTH STUDY - PHS
22,771 subjects were studied to determine the effect of 325mg aspirin daily on cardiovascular mortality. The aspirin group had a slight non fatal risk reduction - less than 1% - and no overall reduction in cardiovascular mortality. Aspirin increased the relative risk of hemorrhagic stroke by 22%.

THROMBOSIS PREVENTION TRIAL - TPT
5,499 men were studied in a placebo controlled trial to evaluate daily aspirin for the prevention of ischemic heart disease. A relative risk reduction of 20% - absolute risk reduction 2.3% - was demonstrated in non fatal myocardial infarctions. However, this came at a cost of a significant increase in hemorrhagic strokes without any decrease in all cause mortality.

THE ANTI PLATLET TRIALISTS COLLOBRATION - ATC
The ATC preformed a meta-analysis of one hundred and forty five randomized studies that sought to use aspirin to decrease

the combined end point of MI, stroke and cardiovascular death. No difference was found between placebo and treated groups.

HYPERTENSION OPTIMAL TRIAL - HOT

With 18,790 participants this trial reported a 15% relative risk reduction for major cardiovascular events. This correlates to an absolute risk reduction of 0.2% per year. There was however, 100% increase in bleeding episodes in the aspirin group and there was no indication of difference in over all mortality.

PRIMARY PREVENTION PROJECT - TPP

4,495 women were studied to evaluate aspirin versus placebo on the occurrences of major cardiovascular events. The primary end point demonstrating cumulative risk of 2.8% in placebo and 2% in the aspirin group. **This corresponds to an absolute risk decrease of 0.2% per year. There was no indication of reduction in total mortality.**

How much meaning and validity can we assign to a decrease in non fatal events of 0.2% per year - or 5 non fatal events per 1000 people treated? **In order to demonstrate how meaningless this data really is, let's do a little trick of our own ----**

The PPT study had cumulative cardiovascular events of 6.3% in the aspirin group and 8.3% in the placebo group in 4495 patients over a period of 42 months. This appears to show a 2% benefit for the aspirin takers. Now let's take some data from a similar study called CHARISMA in 15,603 identical high risk subjects, and substitute the CHARISMA aspirin group for the aspirin group used in the PPT study....

The CHARISMA group on aspirin demonstrated a cumulative total of 7.3% cardiovascular events reached in 28 months. This extrapolates to 11% cumulative total of adverse cardiovascular events that would have been reached at 42 months! The placebo group in the PPT trial was 8.3% at 42 months--- If we

65

now plug in the aspirin group from the Charisma study of 11%.... we now have an overall **absolute risk increase of 2.8% for the subjects on aspirin.** (11% aspirin minus 8.3% placebo) We are just swapping the placebo group results which should not change anything since they are identical high risk groups. **This exercise reversed the result.** It becomes strikingly clear that a 0.2% per year purported difference in risk is far too small to have any meaning what-so-ever, and, simply put- these studies are garbage.

I would again emphasize that the Meta-analyses of large numbers of studies consistently show an approximate 1% increase in over all mortality in subjects on aspirin therapy as opposed to placebo and this, after all, is the most important bottom line.(1% increase in death rate of 50million people over 70 is equal to 50,000 deaths per year!)

If aspirin were to truly have a beneficial effect, this would most surely be demonstrable in subjects at the highest risk level. The highest risk cohorts are subjects with diabetes.

An analysis of three trials utilizing the subset of diabetics demonstrated no difference in cardiovascular death, stroke, MI or total cardiovascular events between the aspirin and placebo groups.

An additional ten thousand studies added to hundreds that have already been done cannot and would not alter the reality that aspirin has not been proven to have saved one single life. However, apparently a lot of people remain desperate to prove something positive about aspirin and cardiovascular disease and I must, therefore, not omit the results of the "long awaited",

WOMEN'S HEALTH STUDY.
39,876 women were randomly allocated to aspirin or placebo for a period of ten years, this study showed no benefit in reduction of major cardiovascular events and no benefit in respect to MI, cardiovascular mortality or total mortality.

66

This should have put an end to this endless exercise in futility, but hold on; headlines blared" study shows 17% reduction in stroke risk for woman on aspirin". This finding was trumpeted by the media as a great step forward, ignoring the fact that the study failed to corroborate any benefits purported to be shown in any previous study for Aspirin. Additionally, no previous study had ever found a decrease in stroke risk in women or in men, in fact, meta- analyses of previous studies on fifty-five thousand subjects showed no benefit for prevention of stroke or cardiac death. A 13% **increase** in over all stroke risk and a disturbing 67% **increase** in the risk of hemorrhagic stroke! Hemorrhagic strokes are far more catastrophic with an 80% initial death rate compared to 10% in ischemic stroke, as well as, 80% long term disability in the survivors of hemorrhagic stroke.

As for the purported 17% decrease of stroke in this study ,if we accept it as real-- as all other studies show otherwise ,this amounts to an absolute reduction of risk of 0.16% per year for stroke with no reduction in over- all mortality. We have previously made it clear that these tiny differences are simply not meaningful or reliable in any clinical trial.

A few years ago I, like many others, decided to try a little experiment. What could it hurt? So, I took my first and only Viagra tablet and waited for the expected result--- no I didn't get the dreaded" over 4 hour side effect"- but I did get major chest pain and a trip to the hospital for a coronary angioplasty and the placing of a coronary artery stent. At this point I had considerable trust in my cardiologist- he seemed quite expert in his field and was a nice guy as well. Of course, he put me on a regimen of aspirin as well as Plavix, an anti-platelet clumping and blood thinning agent.

As we have seen aspirin, at best, does nothing beyond the usual side effects and if we use the data from the PPT and CHARISMA as we have shown previously I now had a 33% increased risk of death. But my cardiologist was not finished-

He had put me on Plavix as well. Now, Plavix happens to be the second largest selling drug in the world, so one would think it was a well proven lifesaver. Hold on!

A recent study published in the New England Journal of Medicine showed that **Plavix increased the overall death risk by 100% when taken long term.** Now my cardiologist had more than doubled my risk of death instead of helping me-- This is the mess doctors have gotten themselves into.

Judging from the objective data, doctors may well be responsible for at least half of all deaths following a cardiac event, not to mention the severe bleeding problems seen commonly with Plavix and the many cases of fatal TTP (thrombotic thrombocytopenic purpura).

Needless to say, I never took either drug. But I did see a great T.V. add recently, extolling the virtues of Plavix as a powerful protection against recurrent heart attack. The ad was so good I almost fell for it myself. The man in the white coat was so reassuring; I hardly even noticed the required iteration of side effects that slid lugubriously from his lips.

As bad as all this looks we have not yet seen the half of it. So far we have found no benefit at all - but what about the risks?

CHAPTER VIII
DAMAGE CONTROL

In the previous chapter, we saw that the highly publicized and long awaited WOMENS HEALTH STUDY found a 67% increase in the risk of hemorrhagic stroke with aspirin treatment - scary enough - but, let's look at some additional data on this issue and the whole subject of the toxicity and side effects of aspirin.

ASPIRIN USE AND THE RISK OF STROKE IN THE ELDERLY; "THE ROTTERDAM STUDY"
Aspirin considerably increased the risk of first time stroke in subjects free from vascular disease. (Relative risk 1.80).

A LANCET published study for the University of Oxford found that in the past 25 years the number of strokes associated with blood thinning agents "primarily aspirin" had risen 7 fold. "The rise is particularly high in the over 75 age group and aspirin may do more harm than good in healthy older people". (Note the ubiquitous use of the word "may" in hedging on negative findings).

Stroke is by no means the only serious adverse event secondary to long term aspirin use. Note the following:

1. Aspirin taken for 20 years increased the risk of pancreatic cancer 58% (survival rate of less than 5%0). (Journal of National Cancer Institute).
2. Long term aspirin therapy results in a 49% increase in cataract formation.
3. Aspirin is the major cause of acid reflux or GERD.
4. 20% of asthma attacks are induced by aspirin.
5. American Journal of Medicine 2003: daily aspirin caused deterioration of kidney function in elderly patients.
6. Aspirin can cause liver damage especially in persons using alcohol.
7. Aspirin increased the incidence of gastrointestinal bleeding; which can be fatal.

Since the best interpretation of aspirin benefit shows a need to treat between 250 and 700 persons for several years to achieve any risk reduction end point, it would be incredible to propose that aspirin would not be responsible for more than a single death or serious adverse advent in such a large and unlucky cohort.

The story doesn't end there even though it should. On the heels of the withdrawal of Bayer's statin drug, Baycol (cerivastatin)due to increasing reports of severe and often fatal rhabdomyolysis (muscle wasting) Bayer now introduces - Bayer aspirin with Heart Advantage - combining aspirin and phytosterols. A new marketing strategy purported to lower cholesterol and also to prevent heart disease and strokes. Apparently Bayer thinks that combining two useless drugs together would be more effective than two useless drugs taken independently.

It should be increasingly apparent that the primary purpose of these excessive numbers of clinical trials is not to add new knowledge to medicine. Their primary purpose is to garner publicity for their sales programs and more importantly to constitute a massive bribe which buys the loyalty of the entire research community, who then become mere surrogates to the marketing strategies of the major drug companies.

A telling case in point which illustrates this thinly disguised "modus operandi" is the story of Merck's Vytorin. The ENHANCE trial compared the effect of the cholesterol drug Vytorin with the effect of Zocor. Vytorin is a combination of the drug Zetia and Zocor. Since Zetia and Zocor use different ways of reducing cholesterol the combination was thought to reduce cholesterol more effectively than Zocor alone. Such a clinical trial is not significant new knowledge but simply an attempt to create another marginally useless product to capture sales from Lipitor.

After a long period of suppression and delay in publishing the results, Merck released the information that

Vytorin [the dual drug] provided no benefit over Zocor alone and indeed caused considerably more arterial plaque buildup than was seen with Zocor. This occurred despite the fact that Vytorin achieved a much greater decrease in cholesterol levels! This was certainly not what was wanted: In order to show that cardiovascular disease is improved by lower cholesterol levels the result had to be the opposite.

The way in which researchers and high- placed medical experts responded to this glaring indication that the entire premise upon which these drugs are based is faulty, was as follows--

Dr. Robert Spiegel, Chief Medical Officer for Merck/Schering said, "the plaque reduction may not have been large because all the participants had already been on cholesterol-lowering statins for many years, which might have already cleaned the plaque out from their arteries". This was the first of many pathetic attempts to blame their own study design for its negative (unwanted) results.

Joining in the damage control was the respected and prestigious Dr. Howard Weintraub, Clinical Director of the Center for the prevention of cardiovascular disease at New York Medical Center and Associate Professor at New York University School of Medicine. Certainly high credentials for someone who's best response was - "ENHANCE found that plaque got slightly worse when the drug combination was used - but, the real take home message here is that getting LDL down is important, and that's not something that should get lost as a consequence of this study".

This statement was made in spite of the fact that researchers for ENHANCE found no difference in heart attack or stroke at the lower cholesterol levels and that Vytorin caused double the build-up of arterial plaque. This rather mindless plea not to abandon a thoroughly discredited hypothesis is simply a testimony to the total enslavement of

72

the medical profession by the never ending flow of dollars from Big Pharma.

Not to be deterred by the Vytorin fiasco, Merck and Schering upped the ante again in their marketing campaign disguised as drug research and initiated a 10,000 patient study to determine whether Vytorin protects against heart attacks, strokes and death better than Zocor alone. Stay tuned for the results of this massive medical break through due in 2011.

It is truly doubtful that the pharmaceutical companies and the research facilities engaged in these exercises would have any interest in a technology not related to the ones they are being paid for. Regardless of the potential benefit which that technology might show. This suppression of alternate and better technology is not merely a theoretical problem.

An important new technology does exist and has been suppressed for many years. There is, however, a little more that you need to know before we get to what may be the most important chapter in this book.

CHAPTER IX
SCRUBBING THOSE PESKY FREE RADICALS

I look forward to the day when a trip to the super market is medicine at its highest level. Tomatoes will have little stickers - your Lycopene by Merck - bananas instead of Chiquita will say potassium courtesy of Pfizer. Antioxidants and vitamins in my cereal by Kellogg's Pharmaceuticals. Immune stimulation in my yogurt courtesy of Dannon/Squib.

On and on, everywhere I look, everything from cereal to cosmetics packed with life saving antioxidants. Food is medicine - medicine is food- all for a healthier and happier life. No more heart disease, no more cancer, no aging. Marketers and consumers have come to a consensus that you can never get enough of a good thing.

Many years ago it was discovered that vitamins can treat and prevent vitamin deficiency diseases - like scurvy, pellagra, rickets, beri-beri and a whole host of vitamin deficiency diseases. Somebody then surmised that vitamins had to be good for a multiplicity of other things too. Nobody cared much that vitamins are neither a food nor even a nutrient. Vitamins are catalysts to enhance biochemical reactions in the body and are therefore only required in very tiny amounts. Amounts easily obtained through a normal diet in the normal person.

But then, along came a very bright man named Linus Pauling who, in the course of his career as a molecular chemist, won two Nobel prizes. Unfortunately, Linus suffered from the same malady as a host of other prominent scientists - he just never could let go of a false hypothesis, no matter what the evidence showed.

If there is one idea in medicine today that is most responsible for the sorry state of modern pharmaceutical medicine and for countless unnecessary deaths, it's Linus Pauling's nonsensical theory of using antioxidants (vitamin C) to scrub those pesky oxygen free-radicals from the body.

A free- radical is a highly reactive atom or molecule that has an unpaired electron in its outer shell and is always looking for an atom or molecule to react with. On the theory that these free radicals, which are produced within our own white blood cells, are toxic and cause everything from arthritis to aging, Linus Pauling decided to flood the body with antioxidants and scrub out all these pesky free radicals, hoping to cure countless diseases, including cancer.

Of course no hypothesis will be allowed to fail if there is money to be made out of it, and the fact is, that after 50 years and thousands of trials no antioxidant has been shown to significantly benefit any human disease. Nevertheless, we are living today in the fabulous age of vitamin and antioxidant mania.

I wonder if anyone ever thought that it would not be a good idea to prevent our immune system from making free radicals when it needs them. It seems a little like advising a patient to remove his offending lymph nodes when they become swollen in the course of disease - or maybe we should bleed him as was done in the good old days to remove some of those free radicals from his body.

Did anyone ever think that dosing a person with antioxidants might not protect his own cells but protect the viruses, bacteria and fungi, which don't have their own antioxidant protection, as our cells do? Free radicals are our body's way of killing invading organisms and destroying toxins. Any treatment which decreases our body's ability to produce free radicals or destroys free radicals can only have the effect of suppressing immune function and increasing our susceptibility to disease, infection and cancer.

As we have seen, anytime a hypothesis becomes a money maker, as in the seven billion dollar a year vitamin business, this hypothesis becomes hardwired into the brains of researchers and academics who, thereafter, seem doomed to repeating the same trials over and over and continuously being puzzled as to the wrong outcomes. To date there have been over eight hundred major clinical trials testing vitamins and/or antioxidants on countless diseases and all- cause mortality - they have all failed - and the recommendation is always the same - more studies need to be done. Vitamins have their uses--but not as anti-oxidants! Beware of A, C and E.

VITAMIN E AND BETA CAROTINE - CANCER PREVENTION STUDY-ATBC

New England Journal of Medicine 1994.

In this study 29,133 subjects were used to determine whether Vitamin E and Vitamin A would reduce the incidence of cancer. In this study the use of beta carotene (vitamin A) showed an 18% increase in lung cancer and an 8% increase in total mortality. Vitamin E showed no beneficial effect and a slight increase in stroke and cancer rates.

BETA CAROTENE AND VITAMIN A ON LUNG CANCER AND CARDIOVASCULAR DISEASE -CARET -

New England Journal of Medicine 1996.

This study was on 18,314 subjects, the effects of vitamin E and vitamin A to determine the effects of a combination of vitamin E and vitamin A on the incidence of lung cancer and death from cardiovascular disease versus placebo. The relative risk of all cause death was increased 17% in the treated group. The risk of death from lung cancer was increased by 46%. The risk from cardiovascular disease was increased 26%. On the basis of these findings, the randomized trial was stopped 21 months earlier than planned.

PHYSICIANS HEALTH STUDY; PHS

No benefit shown with beta carotene.

WOMENS HEALTH STUDY; WHS

No benefit shown with beta carotene and vitamin A.

ARCHIVES OF INTERNAL MEDICINE - META-ANALYSIS 2004

In an analysis of 7 randomized trials - 6 of the 7 trials showed no significant efficacy of vitamin E or vitamin C on cardiovascular disease.

HIGH DOSE VITAMIN E SUPPLEMENTATION - META-ANALYSIS - ANNALS OF INTERNAL MEDICINE - 2005
A metaanalysis 13, 5967 participants in 99 clinical trials was performed. Analysis showed a statistical relationship between vitamin E dosage and increased all-cause mortality at dosages greater than 150 IU / day.

COCHRANE REVIEW - JOURNAL OF AMERICAL MEDICAL ASSOCIATION 2008.
In this analysis all primary and secondary clinical trials of antioxidant supplements (beta carotene, vitamin A, vitamin C, vitamin E and selenium) versus placebo were included. 67 trials with 232,550 subjects were included.
Antioxidants significantly increased all cause mortality between 6% and 18%. A co-author Dr.N.D.Gluud stated "we cannot exclude the possibility that they may be even more harmful if used for longer than the duration of the trials included in our review".

BRITISH MEDICAL JOURNAL 1999 - A meta-analysis of three trials of vitamin C shows an increase in mortality of 8%.

DEPARTMENT OF PUBLIC HEALTH UNIVERSITY OF HELSINKI
60 studies examined the effects of vitamin C on the common cold. No effect was observed in cold incidence in the six largest studies. Vitamin C had no preventative effects in normally nourished subjects in western countries. Regular vitamin C supplementation, in the four largest studies, reduced the duration of colds, but only by 5%. They end with the obligatory statement "further carefully designed trials are needed".

JAMA 2002: EFFECTS OF HORMONE REPLACEMENT AND ANTI-OXIDANT VITAMIN SUPPLEMENTS ON CORONARY ATHEROSCLEROSIS IN POST MENOPAUSAL WOMEN.

Over 2.8 years progression of coronary artery plaque was measured in 423 women. Women on antioxidant vitamins worsened by .044 mm/yr compared to placebo of .028mm/yr or almost **double the progression of coronary artery disease.**

LANCET 2004 METANALYSIS OF 14 TRIALS OF ANTIOXIDANT SUPPLEMENTS

This analysis included 14 trials and 170,000 subjects and showed an increase in mortality for cancers of the stomach, esophagus, large bowel and pancreas. Commenting on these results, David Foreman and Douglas Altman, of the University of Leeds in England stated," The prospect that vitamin pills may not only do no good but also kill their consumers is a scary speculation given the vast quantities that are used."

"Scary speculation" may be the way they see it, but if we are to give some credence to the large study performed at the University of Washington and published in the NEJM (previously mentioned), we see an increase in overall death rate of 18%. It would not be out of line to calculate that this translates to approximately 200,000 deaths per year in the U.S. This would qualify vitamins as the third leading cause of death in America-a scary prospect indeed-but not one that seems to deter the antioxidant express.

An interesting study published in Cell Metabolism 2007 reveals that worms on glucose restriction had an increase of their lifespan of 20%. The worms increased their mitochondrial activity for energy production which led to an increased production of reactive oxygen species (free radicals).Treatment with antioxidant vitamins eliminated the life extending effect. Researchers called the result "scary" because it means that, rather than being protective, antioxidants may actually leave the body more vulnerable by thwarting natural defenses.

I sent a communication to these researchers pointing out that at KEMRI we had shown that free radicals (ALPHAMIR- described in later chapters) provide a significant longevity benefit not associated with glucose or calorie restriction. Of course I never received any reply--it is quite phenomenal how little interest researchers show in the implications of their work, once they move on to their next funded project.

Another study was presented in Experimental Biology by researchers at the University of North Carolina in 2001. Mice with breast cancer that were fed antioxidant free diets had one fourth as many metastases and their tumors shrank by 50% compared to rats on standard diets containing antioxidants.

Finally, a team of researchers from the University College London led by Tony Segal of the center for molecular medicine published a paper in Nature in 2004. **The researchers stated that all the theories relating to the cause of disease by oxygen free- radicals and the therapeutic value of antioxidants must be reevaluated**. The University College London (UCL) categorically discounts the primary evidence upon which this theory is based." white blood cells produce oxygen-free radicals which are essential for the killing of invading microorganisms. Our work shows that the basic theory underlying the toxicity of oxygen free-radicals is flawed".

Continuing to ignore the science, and in the wake of all of these "failed" studies, researchers invariably called for additional studies for further elucidation of the role of antioxidants. One can only marvel as to why the weight of these countless failed trials does not penetrate their consciousness. The untold waste in talent and treasure, over decades, trying to validate useless remedies stands as a callous insult to the millions who die each year from cancer and heart

80

disease, after placing false hope in what never could and never will save one of them.

How many real and effective drugs could have been brought forward if medical science was not channeled and controlled by the profit mongers? As you read these pages countless such studies are finishing and new ones are beginning. The Harvard University Observational trial-87,000 participants, A Harvard study of 40,000 female health professionals, A study in France using a vitamin cocktail on 15,000 healthy men and women- A U.S. study on 160,000 woman on vitamin use and death rates--and the list goes on.

In September 2008 The SELECT study sponsored by the National Cancer Institute and begun in 2001 was stopped early. The study on 35,000 men was to determine the benefit of vitamin E and selenium to prevent prostate cancer. It seems, however, that vitamin E caused an increase in prostate cancer and selenium caused an increase in diabetes. The National Cancer Institute was quick to point out that these findings could be due to chance and participants will continue to be monitored. This kind of disclaimer is never seen when miniscule results are seen in the "right" direction as in the JUPITER trial using Crestor. In that trial a reduction of one tenth of one percent of nonfatal heart attacks in one year was lauded as a major breakthrough in the treatment of heart diseas!.

The SELECT study disappointed many cancer experts, says Elise Cook M.D., a cancer prevention specialist at M.D. Anderson Cancer Center in Houston. Cook says many men had been reluctant to join the study because they were already taking vitamin E for heart as well as prostate health. "Since then, other studies have shown that it didn't really help their hearts either."

In the midst of this immense tempest in a teapot, endlessly revisiting useless and failed studies ,it would be perhaps permissible to wonder why new ideas and approaches are forever eschewed by the interlocked research institutes and pharmaceutical giants that decide what to study and what to dispense. It certainly is not that alternative life- saving technologies are not put forward, as we will soon see.

Meanwhile, doctors have relegated themselves to the intellectual level of chimpanzees. They are lucky to have white coats to cover their hairy bodies and plastic surgeons to pin back their protruding ears. I will temporize on that statement, somewhat, since there certainly are many wonderful doctors, who are skilled surgeons or practitioners, and who care about the lives of their patients. But even these have to bear the fiduciary burden of failing to open their eyes to what is going on around them because they feel too overwhelmed with their busy lives and practices.

The seriousness of this appalling level of dogma and intransigence cannot be over-estimated. Beyond the mountain of data and the myriad of clinical trials there is an even more telling proof of the failure of these hypotheses and, more importantly, it is a technological breakthrough that threatens to change the world of medicine forever. For that story you will have to journey with me through the odyssey of Doctor D.

CHAPTER X
A DOCTOR'S ODYSSEY

Dr. D. had recently retired from practice. Still young at only 50 -- He had just gone through surgery to remove several nodules. The path report told the story, malignant lymphoma. Within a few weeks one of the nodules began to grow again so local radiation (5000 rads) was done to the area.

A year later Dr. D's stepson turned up with a small purple lesion on his face - 28 years old and openly gay, but a sweet, happy- go- lucky kid who everybody loved. Of course it was the worst possible news; it was Kaposi's sarcoma, a tumor associated with full blown AIDS. The young man had lived for a while in San Francisco and had participated in a massive gay rally heralding a new era for gay rights. Little did they know that this event foreshadowed a coming holocaust.

The year was 1978 and along with many of his friends he was convinced by a poster advertising a protective vaccine for hepatitis B that was now available for active homosexual men. The poster stated that following this trial the vaccine would not be available for anyone for several years. So he along with several thousand other members of the San Francisco gay community presented themselves for injection with the new hepatitis B vaccine. (We shall return to this event in a later chapter).

Following the diagnosis of AIDS on his stepson Ken, Dr. D made a promise to him that he would do everything in his power to keep him alive until a cure was found. So Dr. D began an odyssey to many major university research facilities and talked to many researchers - experts in the field of infectious diseases. The truth was quickly apparent. It was 1985 and there was not only no effective treatment for AID's, but there was no foreseeable breakthrough expected for at least 10 years. The best they had to offer was chemotherapy borrowed from cancer treatments. As life expectancy with AID's at that time did not exceed 24 months, it was clearly an absolute death sentence for the growing number of gay young men presently infected.

Dr. D. was unenthusiastic about the rationale for treating a viral infection with chemotherapy -- there had to be

84

a better way. If there was one thing he knew for certain it was that a normal immune system could cope with the vast majority of viral infections and ultimately control or eliminate the virus. If a white blood cell can kill a virus perhaps it would be possible to augment its killing power by providing more of what the normal white cell uses. Dr. D. thought that this could be a shortcut way to delay the inevitable in those now under sentence of death.

White blood cells kill viruses by producing a high energy bio-oxidant called super-oxide -- therefore, Dr. D. decided he would look for a way to synthesize a molecular structure which would release super-oxide and augment the ability of the immune system to fight a virus.

Following considerable research into the chemistry of super-oxide - a highly reactive free-radical - Dr. D. set to work. He purchased some equipment and set up a small laboratory in his guest house and began the process of trying to synthesize a molecular structure which would hold oxygen in a high energy, but stable, state until introduced into an aqueous environment. After six months and over 200 failed attempts, Dr. D. succeeded in creating a special ring structure- a Trioxolane- which would release oxygen as super-oxide.

Now, oxygen comes in many forms besides as the O_2 that we breathe. Super-oxide is O_2 minus, with a missing electron making it a highly reactive free-radical, having the oxidizing power 10,000 times that of stable O_2. This is exactly what he needed to kill viruses - and many other things as well.

Now, it is accepted scientific dogma that oxygen - free radicals are highly toxic and are not considered suitable for therapy. It seemed to Dr. D. that the fact that white blood cells produce free radicals in our own defense, suggested that they might not be nearly as toxic to normal cells as everyone seemed to think - and he was right.

Dr. D. proceeded to inject a group of white mice with huge amounts of his super-oxide producing material using hundreds of times what would be an effective human dose - and sure enough the mice showed no signs of distress or toxicity. The concern about free radical toxicity looked again like a failed hypothesis. Encouraged by this, Dr. D. commissioned a local toxicology laboratory to perform a series of toxicity and antimicrobial tests. Again no toxicity was observed and the compound demonstrated major antimicrobial activity against viruses, bacteria, fungi and protozoa.

Feeling that the time had come to get help in the furtherance of his research, Dr. D. revisited many of the researchers that he had previously seen and some new ones as well, hoping to elicit some interest or curiosity in the academics about a new formulation that had been shown to be broadly antimicrobial and non -toxic. Well, take a guess---- not a single academic had the slightest interest in pursuing this new technology or in assisting Dr. D. in any way.

Since the advent of AID's, Dr's and academics that were previously known as "allergists", had now been promoted to "immunologists" with all the new found celebrity provided by the life and death struggle against AID's. Basking in the limelight of frequent news and television interviews and fortified by huge money and innumerable new projects from Big Pharma, they simply had no time or interest in an upstart doctor with no research credentials.

Arriving home one day after a fruitless sojourn to his old alma mater, the University Of Southern California School Of Medicine, Dr. D. found a handsome young man waiting for him on his doorstep. The young man introduced himself - his name was Scott - and proceeded to tell him that he had heard from a friend, a chemical supply salesman, that Dr. D. was working on a new experimental drug for the treatment of AID's. Scott told him, that he had tried everything one could imagine, but he was continuing to deteriorate from AID's. Scott was a concert pianist and found that he could no longer play. He was having severe cognitive loss and was willing to try anything. He asked Dr. D. to consider him as a candidate for use of this experimental drug. This was a startling request for Dr. D. because he had not as yet considered the option of testing the drug on humans himself - and besides as he told Scott - The long-term toxicology studies which were underway had not yet been completed. And so he sent Scott away.

One week later two things happened, Dr. D. was again rebuffed by several more academic researchers in his quest for assistance and a new nodule had formed at the edge of his radiation site. In the mist of this there was a knock at his door and there stood Scott, the young pianist who wanted to be the first test case and wouldn't take no for an answer. He was getting worse and was willing and anxious to take any risk. Thus began Dr. D's journey with Scott into a world that neither would have imagined.

Scott was sent to a lab to obtain his baseline blood work and the next day he presented himself, after a short visit to his church, at Dr. D's house for his first treatment. The initial treatment was given intravenously and started at a very low dose and was increased daily until the dosage that Dr. D. calculated was sufficient was reached. Following the first few treatments and as all was progressing without a problem, Dr. D. began injecting himself as well.

Thirty days later, repeat laboratory tests showed no evidence of toxicity and Scott's T-4 cell level (the white blood cells that the AID'S virus attacks) went from 190 to a level of 1200. This was unheard in the entire history of AID's - and for good measure, the recurrent tumor on Dr. D's chest had disappeared.

These results encouraged Dr. D. to open a small study to a few more AID's patients and he was soon able to recruit a group of ten. All were fully informed that the study involved an experimental non- approved drug, according to the Helsinki Declaration which outlined procedures necessary for any human study not sanctioned by an academic institutional review board. In addition, FDA rules clearly allowed a licensed physician to use his best judgment in these matters for the treatment of patients, particularly in the instance of fatal disease,

I will be as succinct as possible to compress a long story into a brief synopsis. In the ensuing 2 years data was collected on these 10 patients. All had major clearing of symptoms and their T-4 cell levels increased from an average of 250 to 750. Of course academics continued to show no interest and discounted the value of the data, however positive, on such a small number of patients.

Toward the end of 1989, one of Dr. D's patients was doing so well that he took it upon himself to call an AIDS hotline (Project Inform) and tell one of their executives about the success of this new treatment. The response of Martin Delaney of Project Inform was to immediately contact the State Attorney General and report that a doctor was treating AID's patients with an unapproved drug and to importune them to intervene and stop him. (Certainly one would have to wonder what motivated a pro AID's group to take this action; however, I will tell you that this was indeed the attitude of all so called AIDS groups, including AMFAR and Act Up).

Dr. D. was subsequently charged by the State Attorney Generals Office with a misdemeanor health and safety code violation - that is -using a non FDA approved treatment for AID's. Ultimately these charges were expunged by stipulation of the judge, based on the efficacy of the treatment.

In addition to this, an attorney named Ray Henke recruited one of Dr. D's patients and promised him a five million dollar windfall payoff if he would sue Dr. D. for malpractice. One would have to wonder who was financing this suit as this attorney ultimately spent more than a million dollars pursuing it. During the course of this civil suit, the plaintiff, whose name, appropriately enough, was Looney, signed a written statement repudiating everything that he had charged against Dr. D. and stating that he had been convinced to perjure himself by attorney Henke. At the end of a long drawn out trial, the judge threw out the case and charged Looney with perjury and attorney Henke with subornation of perjury and declared the whole affair to be a conspiracy to extort money.

Of course, not unexpectedly, the Medical Board regarded the use of Dr. D's right, as a licensed physician, to treat these patients as he saw fit, with horror and indignation-- going so far as to liken it to Nazi experiments on concentration camp inmates. As if that was not enough, they then proceeded to demonstrate a level of ignorance almost unprecedented in scientific circles by charging that Dr.D. was injecting his patients with lemon juice. They then expressed puzzlement over where he got the idea that lemon juice could be anti-viral.

In spite of this incredible harassment, Dr. D. presented remarkable data on ten patients at the International AID's Conference in San Francisco in 1990. As part of his presentation, all of the patients gathered at a nearby hotel, anxious to be interviewed by any of the conference participants who might be interested in this new technology and how well they were doing.

Of course, Scott was there and as it happened one of his closest friends, a doctor who worked at the National Institute of Health, was in the room directly across the hall. When Scott asked him to come over to see the group of AIDS patients that were gathered, he hurriedly backed off and said "Scott- don't come near me again - do you want me to lose my job?" Needless to say, Scott never again heard from his ex-lover.

The general response to Dr. D's presentation was no better. With great hostility Doctor after doctor questioned the veracity of his data and implied that he had rigged the numbers, as they were far more impressive than anything they had been able to accomplish.

The conference was a conclave of AIDS bigwigs; all sponsored by major drug companies, and all basking in the exalted stature that AIDS was affording them. Certainly, a "medical nobody" was not going to be allowed to cast a shadow on their new-found luminosity.

Despite this negativity, Dr. D. did meet one academician who expressed genuine interest and out of that meeting Dr. D. received an invitation to come and work on his technology at the Kenya Medical Research Institute (KEMRI) in Nairobi, Kenya. The Kenya Medical Research Institute is the eighth largest research institute in the world and had the will and the capacity to prove once and for all the value of "Trioxolane Technology". Thus Dr. D. took a position as Chief Director of Research at KEMRI and set off for Nairobi.

What came out of Africa might surprise you.

CHAPTER XI
OUT OF AFRICA

Dr. D. arrived in Nairobi at the main campus of KEMRI. Working together with many staff members, Dr. D. was determined to prove that Trioxolane was a better way, despite the indifference of the scientific community. The history of medicine is filled with failed hypotheses and failure to recognize failure, as well as, failure to recognize new successes.

One of the most important discoveries in the history of medicine was made serendipitously by Sir Alexander Fleming. Some Petri dishes that had not yet been cleaned were left on his window sill and it happened that airborne mold spores had contaminated them. A substance produced by the mold could be seen inhibiting the growth of bacteria around them. Thus penicillin was discovered in 1928.

As was the wont of medical experts, the discovery seemed to have little significance to them and lay dormant for nearly 15 years. At the outbreak of the Second World War, in a desperate search for some solutions to the problem of gas gangrene infection, a major cause of death in World War One, two academics came upon a long forgotten publication about the penicillin mold. With this in hand they approached The British War Ministry and asked for funds to develop a method to grow the spores and extract the penicillin. Of course, they were turned down, but the era of antibiotics was born.

The impact of antibiotics on the treatment of bacterial disease was, as we know, revolutionary. Unfortunately, we now may be witnessing the beginning of the end of the era of antibiotics, as the emergence of antibiotic resistant organisms becomes an ever increasing problem. In light of this, it is all the more perplexing as to why the medical profession is indifferent to new antimicrobial technology. Even more puzzling is the absence of interest in a true broad spectrum antiviral agent, since medicine has not as yet found such a creature, and remains devoid of any truly effective treatment for viral disease.

Medicine's approach to the treatment of viral disease has been almost exclusively through the use of vaccines and it appears that the huge financial success of vaccine programs has led to diffidence about the need for an effective antiviral agent. More and more vaccines are being produced, and are in the pipeline, to augment what has become a hugely profitable industry. (We will get into vaccines in another chapter).

A basic hypothesis being put forward by Dr. D. in the utilization of Trioxolane was that immune stimulation, rather than immune suppression, was a superior way to treat disease. One of the primary dogmas of modern medicine is the belief that so -called "auto-immune" disease is caused by over-stimulation of our own immune system causing our immune system to attack our own tissues. The prototypical autoimmune disease is rheumatoid arthritis. There are many others such as: lupus, scleroderma, diabetes, colitis - the list is long. Based on this hypothesis, autoimmune disease is invariably treated with immuno-depressant drugs such as: steroids, monoclonal antibodies (to attack and destroy white blood cells) and chemotherapy. Unfortunately, this doesn't work very well and destroying the immune system is probably a bad idea as it leads to severe side effects, infections and cancer. Never-the-less, as in most medical dogmas, doctors are far from ready to abandon a bad hypothesis.

The reader might be wondering what all this has to do with Dr. D. and Trioxolane. I can assure you it does, as we shall discover shortly.

It is well known that free radicals do many things in our body - they kill invading organisms, they stimulate immune function and they kill tumor cells. So why should they cause "autoimmune" disease? Well, just like previous hypotheses that have been shown to be wrong, Dr. D. came to the conclusion that the entire theory of autoimmune disease was backward and that immune stimulation would be of more benefit that immune suppression. If he was right Trioxolane could not only be a potent antiviral for the treatment of AID's, hepatitis and influenza, but would be effective in rheumatoid arthritis and other autoimmune diseases. Additionally super-oxide as a potent tumor cell killer would be a useful adjunct to both cancer therapy and would prevent immune system depression during chemotherapy. Lastly, he surmised that since super-oxide has been utilized by mammalian immune systems as an antimicrobial for millions of years, it was extremely unlikely that any organism could become resistant to treatment with Trioxolane.

So how close to the truth was Dr. D. -- would Trioxolane emerge from Africa as a major contribution to medicine or was he chasing an illusion? Up to now all of his efforts have been ridiculed and disparaged by the best minds in American medicine. Well, let's see the data :

In the first year at KEMRI Dr. D. supervised a program of in-vitro antimicrobial testing, animal toxicity studies and in-vivo animal studies. The results of these tests were published as following:

TRIOXOLANES - A NEW GENERATION OF COMPOUNDS WITH WIDE RANGING ACTIVITIES - AFRICAN JOURNAL OF HEALTH SCIENCE 1994.

INVITRO ACTIVITY

Direct activity of Trioxolane was accessed in-vitro using cells, protozoa, bacteria and fungi. It was shown that Trioxolane was more active than conventional drugs against a broad spectrum of commonly encountered micro- organisms. These micro- organisms were uniformly sensitive to Trioxolane and the activity of the product on these micro-organisms had no relationship with their resistance and sensitivity to conventional antibiotics.

At dilutions of less than: $1: 2 \times 16$ to -10 a myeloma (tumor) cell line was killed within 48 hours.

Human spermatozoa were killed within 1 minute at dilutions of 1 to 2000.

Oral LD 50 (measure of toxicity) was 5000mg/kg - that is, non- toxic.

Intra peritoneal LD 50 was 600mg/kg - that is, non- toxic. Trioxolane was superior to pentostam in treating leishmania major infection in mice.

Immunomodulatory activity: bone marrow examination of mice on Trioxolane compared to controls revealed significant increase in new clones of lymphocytes, an indication of major immunostimulatory activity

Conclusion: Trioxolane is anti- microbial, anti- viral, anti-protozoal, Immunomodulatory, spermicidal and tumoricidal. The product is of clinical importance in considering new avenues in the treatment of autoimmune disorders and symptoms associated with HIV infections and AID's.

All of these findings were welcome corroboration of Dr. D's. belief in the correctness of his hypotheses and of the potential importance of this technology. Never-the- less, the medical world remained unimpressed. Dr. D. was indeed bucking an impenetrable and closed system. So he moved on-- feeling certain that, with perseverance, he would reach a break-through point.

At KEMRI two clinical trials were organized; one for Dr. D's first priority, AIDS, and a second clinical trial to test Trioxolane on patients with rheumatoid arthritis.

EFFICACY OF TRIOXLANE IN THE CLINICAL MANAGEMENT OF HIV SEROPOSITIVE AND SYMPTOMATIC INDIVIDUALS -KEMRI
The result of a 12 week study of symptomatic HIV patients versus control were as follows:

T-cell levels in the treated group increased from 556 to 1221 and in the control group decreased from 542 to 479.

Clinical complaints in the treated group decreased from 9.5 to 0 and in the control group decreased from 9.5 to 8.6

The treated group had an average weight gain of 2.2kg compared to 0 for the control group.

The white blood count of the treated group increased from 3.5 to 5.5 compared to the control group which decreased from 3.5 to 3.2.

No toxicity or adverse events were seen.

DETERMINATION OF EFFICACY AND SAFETY OF TRIOXOLANE IN THE MANAGEMENT OF PATIENTS WITH RHEUMATOID ARTHRITIS - KEMRI

A total of 60 patients with rheumatoid arthritis were treated using Trioxolane 200mg daily, sublingually, for 12 weeks. The results were assessed as follows:
   49 subjects showed complete remission.
   8 subjects showed moderate remission
   1 subject showed noticeable improvement
   2 subjects showed no change.
No adverse effects were seen.

A SERIES OF PILOT CLINICAL STUDIES TO ASSESS THE BROAD SPECTRUM POTENTIAL OF TRIOXOLANE: KEMRI

10 patients were treated with topical Trioxolane for oral candidiasis. All infections cleared within 5 days.

5 females were treated with a vaginal preparation of Trioxolane daily for 5 days for vaginal candidiasis with complete clearing of infection. No further treatment was required.

3 patients with lymphoma and 1 with cancer of the base of the tongue were treated with Trioxolane concomitant with chemo and/or radiation therapy. All patients maintained a white count above 4000 throughout treatment and all were tumor free at end of their course of trearment.

30 patients with fungal infections of the skin were treated with a 2% solution of Trioxolane twice daily for 4 to 6 weeks with complete clearing of lesions.

17 Patients with pharyngitis were treated with a 3% solution of Trioxolane 3 times daily. There was complete resolution of symptoms in all patients within 48 to 72 hours.

Following these trials and in consideration of the excellent therapeutic response without evidence of toxicity, the pharmacy and poisons board of the Ministry of Health of the Republic of Kenya (equivalent to US FDA) approved Trioxolane for sale in Kenya for the treatment of rheumatoid arthritis, auto-immune disease and AID's. The official name was now "ALPHAMIR".

Subsequent to its approval Alphamir has been used in the following conditions in a sufficient number of patients to be strongly indicative of its efficacy: hepatitis, multiple sclerosis, colds/influenza, colitis, osteoarthritis, lupus, scleroderma, Guillain-Barre syndrome, asthma, lymphoma, immuno-stimulation during chemotherapy and innumerable topical uses including: acne, herpes, fungal infection, eczema, joint pain, scar prevention , antisepsis and burns.

Alphamir has been shown to increase micro-capillary circulation by prevention of cellular clumping. This strongly suggests a role in prevention of diabetic side effects as well as adverse cardio-vascular events.

Dr. D. was right--- antioxidants and immunosuppressive drugs were inappropriate and immune stimulation works far better for autoimmune disease! While we are on the subject of failed medical hypotheses, and we have already plowed through a lot of them, there is another one that Dr. D. has pointed out that I should mention here. The legacy of the old-time "snake oil" salesmen is the ingrained belief that one drug cannot treat a multitude of conditions. This turns logic on its head. The human immune system does just that- it treats every disease and invading organism the same way-and if we follow what it is telling us we can find a technology with a similar broad spectrum. On the other hand if we continue to believe that we must have a different chemical for every different disease we will be searching in sea urchins and jungle plants for the next hundred years for toxic chemicals that have little affinity for the human body.

If the previous chapters have revealed anything, it is that the general perception of the success of modern medicine is greatly exaggerated, and it is not in our interest to allow new and promising approaches to be ignored by those looking to protect their cash flow. Today's medical failure is tomorrow's pandemic and smug complacency precedes catastrophe.

At this point one would expect some expression of interest from academia, drug companies, doctors, AID's groups, etc. But complacency still reigned and the door was still locked. Millions of dollars flooding into the system, particularly to highly placed African politicians, seems to be impossible to overcome. This money, from the Global Fund and the World Health Organization, as well as the pharmaceutical combine, creates an unbroken phalanx of people unwilling to back away from the strict policies set up by the World Health Organization.

As for the U.S., no technology not emanating from a drug company with all the cash flow that that entails, will be given consideration - proven or not.

If you remember his first patient from 1988 - Scott - you might be interested to know that he is alive and well today, with a healthful appearance belying his 28th year of living with AID's. Unfortunately, Dr. D's stepson died in 1986, just a few months prior to the first synthesis of Alphamir, along with the countless others who failed to survive that decade.

In the ongoing tragedy of AIDS, where 10,000 human beings are dying each day and 15,000 people are infected each day, it is staggering to realize that a technology that provides a safe and effective treatment could be ignored. There is something terribly wrong with a medical system which routinely provides useless and dangerous drugs but has the audacity to contribute to the suppression of lifesaving drugs.

Recently a major study was undertaken to test a substance as a vaginal prophylaxis to prevent transmission of HIV. This multi-million dollar study was financed by a very large and well known philanthropic foundation whose stated priorities include HIV treatment and prophylaxis. Not unexpectedly, the study was a failure, as the substance being tested was seaweed. (One would have to wonder what they were thinking) This same foundation refused to consider KEMRI's request for a small fund to continue research on Trioxolane. The foundations reply stated that other priorities made it impossible for them to consider Trioxolane -- despite the fact that they had just spent more than what was asked for on the failed seaweed study. Now it was made clear that not only had Trioxolane proven effective in AIDS treatment, but had also been formulated into a contraceptive vaginal gel to prevent transmission of HIV. Additionally Trioxolane had proven effective as an anti- malarial and was effective against organisms resistant to all other antibiotics. Even though the foundation had declared all of these issues to be of their highest priority, there just did not seem to be enough left over from their eighty billion dollar fund to address KEMRI's needs.

If all of this seems difficult to understand it would behoove us to look a little further into the true efficacy of the cornucopia of drugs that you see advertised on your television everyday. Let's measure the value of the countless billions of dollars worth of drugs being sold to a gullible public. Is it

99

possible that efficacy is entirely immaterial to drug sales and promotion? Then we will hear more about Alphamir. The world of drugs is a world away from what you think it is.

CHAPTER XII
THE MIND GAME

Just how does a drug company get people to spend billions of dollars on a drug that doesn't work, has serious toxicity, is based on a failed hypothesis and is physically addictive? The proto-typical class of drugs to demonstrate the "modus operandi" or the pattern which they follow is the ever growing gaggle of anti- depressants that have been foisted upon America. Thirty million people are taking SSRI's (selective serotonin reuptake inhibitors). Sales of drugs like Prozac, Paxil, and Lexapro have topped 19 billion dollars per year. 70% of that total is U.S. sales which must make us the most depressed people in the world. How did all of this happen?

First let's examine the hypothesis upon which use of this entire class of drugs is based. The hypothesis simply is that "depression" is the result of a chemical imbalance in the brain - namely low levels of serotonin. Thus a drug which increases of serotonin should work as an "antidepressant". There are two glaring problems with this hypothesis. First there is no credible scientific evidence that serotonin deficiency is linked to any depressive disorder or that an increase in serotonin levels alleviates any mental disorder. Secondly these drugs (SSRI's) simply do not work better than placebo or any other drug which does not affect serotonin levels. There simply is no such thing as a scientifically established balance of serotonin in the brain. So we are again left only with a failed hypothesis underlying a multi million dollar, direct to the consumer, television ad campaign.

The methodology used by drug companies is simply to perform a series of generally flawed and poorly conducted clinical trials - publishing only the ones that show a slight (statistically significant) positive effect over placebo. As we shall see none of the so called" positive result trials" would qualify in the mind of any objective person as clinically significant.

Amazingly, as each new and improved drug is compared against the former state of the art antidepressant, the former drug shows no efficacy over placebo! That process

101

will be seen as we follow Elavil morphing into Prozac, being succeeded by Paxil, followed by Celexa and finally to the state of the art- Lexapro. Here is an example:

2004 LEXAPRO SUPERIOR TO PLACEBO AND PAXIL IN THE TREATMENT OF GENERAL ANXIETY DISORDER.

In a twelve week study [submitted to FDA] comparing Lexapro to placebo and Paxil the following conclusion was stated: "Lexapro had a significantly better therapeutic effect than either placebo or Paxil. **The remission rate at week 12 for Paxil was not significantly higher than placebo.** As Paxil, to a large extent, has been considered to be a standard treatment for many anxiety disorders this further emphasizes the strong results in favor of Lexapro". So now we are being told that Paxil which was supposed to be better than Prozac is no better than placebo. Is it possible that the researchers in this study are completely unaware of the implication of their conclusion?

If we are to accept their conclusion somebody has spent 15 billion dollars a year on drugs no better than placebo. Luckily, we have now found one that is superior to them all. But, are we able to trust in their conclusion of the improved effectiveness of Lexapro?

It should be mentioned that GlaxoSmithKline the makers of Paxil published the results of only one of five trials studying the effect of Paxil on children. That single study showed mixed results. The others not only failed to show any benefit but demonstrated children taking paxil are more likely to become suicidal. GSK is also now facing criminal action in the UK for failing to inform British Safety Regulators about the suicide risk associated with Seroxat (Paxil). The British Regularity Agency (MHRA) banned giving Seroxat to children under 18 and the US FDA issued a similar advisory.

A similar deception was perpetrated by Pfizer who concealed evidence about the safety and efficacy of their antidepressant Zoloft. Only one out of five of their clinical trials indicated superiority over placebo. With that kind of track record it's hard to put much faith in any clinical trial that purports to show efficacy for this class of drugs. But let's look at what the studies say about the state of the art Lexapro, as well as Paxil and Prozac:

IN A DOUBLE BLIND MULTI CENTER STUDY OF PAXIL, NORPRAMIN (TRICYCLIC ANTIDEPRESSANT) OR PLACEBO IN PATIENTS WITH MAJOR DEPRESSION - JOURNAL OF CLINICAL PSYCHOLOGY
The results were as follows:
Mean changes in total HAM-D and CGI-S (measurements of depression) scores from baseline at the 6 week endpoint for **paxil and norpramin were not significantly different than those for the placebo treated groups.**

A DOUBLE BLIND STUDY OF PROZAC VERSUS PLACEBO IN OUTPATIENTS WITH MAJOR DEPRESSION - ANNALS OF CLINICAL PSYCHIATRY 1988
Results: **"there were no significant differences among the treated groups and placebo** in baseline and endpoint depression and anxiety severity, as well as in the degree of depression and anxiety improvement".

As to the new kid on the block - Lexapro:
A DOUBLE BLIND RANDOMIZED TRIAL OF LEXAPRO VERSUS PLACEBO
Concluded: **"there were no significant differences in the treated and the placebo group"**

The department of clinical pharmacology at Sahigrens University Hospital in Sweden had this to say about Lexapro: "on the evidence available to us, the manufacturers claim for the superiority of escitalopram (Lexapro) over citalopram (Celexa) are unwarranted". The Swedish and Danish Drug Regulatory Authorities reached similar conclusions.

Eli Lilly entered the depression sweepstakes in 2004 with its drug Cymbalta. Cymbalta was to be an improved serotonin- nor- epinephrine reuptake inhibitor (SNRI) for treatment of anxiety disorders and other indications. The rationale behind the development of Cymbalta (and Effexor and Prestiq) was that if the inhibition of reuptake of serotonin was good then the additional inhibition of reuptake of norepinephrine would be even better. This turned out to be one more failed medical hypothesis. In a comparative meta-analysis of multiple clinical trials Cymbalta was no better than SSRI's. A head to head comparison of Cymbalta with Lexapro found Cymbalta to be both less tolerable and less effective. (This means that Cymbalta had to be worse than placebo!)

In 2004 the British Medical Journal published findings of the Royal College of Psychiatry's Research Unit in London which analyzed published and unpublished clinical trial data for each antidepressant medication. They had this to say, "in discussing their own data, the authors of all of the four larger studies have exaggerated the benefits and downplayed the harm, or both. Improvement in control [placebo] groups is strong; additional benefits from the drugs are of doubtful clinical significance and adverse effects have been downplayed".

Two weeks after the BMJ article, Lancet published a systematic review of SSRI's for childhood depression that also compared published and unpublished data. When the researchers analyzed the published and unpublished data together, the SSRI's no longer held a reasonable benefit for pediatric depression to justify the apparent risks. There was not a "massive difference between the published materials versus the unpublished but the profile certainly switches from a favorable risk/ benefit ratio to an unfavorable one" the researchers said. And with each of the SSRI's the researchers examined, they found the same trend; the published data was significantly more favorable than the data that had not been peer reviewed.

PLOS MEDICINE 2008: US AND UK RESEARCHERS LED BY IRVING KIRSCH OF HULL UNIVERSITY, UK, STUDIED ALL CLINICAL TRIALS SUBMITTED TO THE FDA FOR THE LICENSING FOR THE FOUR SSRI'S: FLUOXETINE (PROZAC), VENLAFAXINE, NEFAZODONE, PAROXETINE).

They conclude that, "compared with placebo, the new - generation anti depressants do not produce clinically significant improvements in depression in patients who initially have moderate or even very severe depression".

The preceding results should close the argument as to whether SSRI's provide any real or significant clinical benefits in the vast majority of the more than 30 million users in the US. But that doesn't mean that there is not a serious price to pay. There have been recorded a multiplicity of serious side effects - the full list would cover many pages, but I will spare you that and mention only a few.

. Firstly, all SSRI's have serious withdrawal problems. Attempting to stop the drugs, even for one day leads to a host of cognitive, gastrointestinal, cardiac and musculo-skeletal symptoms, as well as increased anxiety and panic attacks. This is the primary reason that people believe that these drugs work, because they feel so miserable and anxious when they try to stop. This is the primary reason that drug companies have no concern that the drugs don't work, because they know that once on them you can't stop: and the massive cash flow from 30 million unsuspecting anti-depressant drug junkies continues.

It is entirely unconscionable that these incredibly addictive and useless drugs are handed out like so much candy to children by doctors who wouldn't dream of giving an addictive opiate to a dying and suffering cancer patient-- because he might become dependent.

The adverse reactions and side effects listed for lexapro, each affecting over 5% of users, include: nausea, insomnia, fatigue and decreased libido. More serious adverse reactions include: increased suicidality, pulmonary hypertension in newborns and a fatal "serotonin syndrome" if the user takes a tryptan drug for migraine headaches. The side effects for the SNRI's are even worse.

A more personal and dramatic portrayal of the real meaning of all this is seen in the following interview of an angry psychiatrist by journalist Jon Rappaport:

"For the past two years, I have been receiving communications from a practicing American psychiatrist, who has an office in the southeastern US. He sees patients privately. Increasingly, this man has been expressing doubts about the drugs he has been prescribing.

Now he has blown the lid off his own profession, and it appears he is ready to switch careers or become an alternative health practitioner.

Here is an excerpt from our recent conversation.
Q: Why do you doubt the psychiatric drugs?
A: They're toxic and injurious.
Q: Which ones?
A: All of them.
Q: And in particular?
A: The antidepressants. Paxil, Prozac, Zoloft, and so on. They are not showing, on balance, good results, and patients have been experiencing adverse effects.
Q: Such as?
A: Sleeplessness, nightmares, erratic behavior, highs and lows, crashes, attempts to commit suicide, exacerbated depression, violence, dramatic personality changes.
Q: Why do you think this is happening?
A: To be honest, I don't know. But my sense is, in general, that the drugs interfere in unpredictable ways with various neurotransmitter systems. I also believe they can work extreme changes in blood sugar levels and electrolyte levels.
Q: Have you tried to communicate your concerns to colleagues and medical groups?

A: For a short time, I did. But I was given the cold shoulder. I got the distinct feeling I was being treated like some wayward child who had his facts all wrong.

Q: Who do you blame for this drugging catastrophe?

A: At the moment, everybody. The doctors, the drug companies, the FDA, the psychiatric teaching institutions, even the press. And at some point, patients are going to have to take responsibility and not follow the orders of their doctors.

Q: Do you believe that doctors should cut back and give the drugs to some people and not others?

A: That sounds good, but there is no way to know what effects the drugs will cause in any given individual, especially as time passes. Even in the short term, I have seen some frightening things.

Q: Do you believe the profession of psychiatry has made some kind of overarching deal with the drug companies?

A: Yes. The drug companies are everywhere. They stick their noses into everyone's business.

Q: what lies about the drugs have you had to purge from your own mind?

A: The main one is that they're some kind of miracle breakthrough. Another one is that I can rely on the judgments and certifications of the FDA. We're playing Russian roulette out here. It's a very dangerous situation.

Q: How about the diagnosis of depression itself?

A: I've come to realize that you can't do an interview with a patient and then come out with a shorthand assessment. It's wrong. It reduces all sorts of problems down to a label, and then you have your official gateway into drugs.

Q: Your colleagues think you're over-reacting?

A: I think I'm under reacting. I think we have an epidemic on our hands, but it has nothing to do with mental disorders. It has to do with the chemicals we're facilitating.

Q: You're saying the science behind the antidepressants is false.

A: Absolutely. Judging by the effects of drugs, it has to be. It may sound good and proper. All the right words are used. But I don't care about that anymore. I go by results. My eyes have been opened.

Q: Then why are the drug companies pushing these drugs?

A: I'm not an expert to speak about that. Certainly there is the profit motive. But I think there is also the myth of progress.

Q: What do you mean?

A: That myth states that technology must keep making advances. It's the legend of forward motion. If technology is to be seen as good, it has to keep turning out better advances---otherwise something is wrong. And there can't be anything wrong.

Q: What are your thoughts about all the revelations of cheating and lying in medical-drug studies?

A: I blame them as well. If they really wanted to, they could police what comes into them more carefully. They could publicize cheaters. They could blackball them. But drug advertisers keep some of these journals afloat.

Q: So vows of ethical behavior on the part of the journals?

A: Half-truths and lies.

Q: If you can't believe the journals...

A: I believe my patients. I listen to them. I work with them, not on them. I trust my own observations.

Q: Do you prescribe psychiatric drugs?

A: Never"

Just off the presses a new study published in the LANCET showed that anti-psychotic drugs such as Risperdal, Thorazine and Stelazine doubled the death risk in the elderly!

During the course of writing this chapter I, at last, was able to convince my wife and daughter to wean themselves off Lexapro, an SSTI, that both had taken for a number of years. Both had protested that without their pills they would be "basket cases" and impossible to live with. After many weeks of severe withdrawal both had markedly less anxiety --and the

constant headaches which my wife had suffered for years disappeared.

No matter how slick the television ads, the pharmaceutical industry cannot escape from the results of their own clinical trials, and as bad as all of this looks, there is far worse to come.

CHAPTER XIII
BONES AND JOINTS

One of the luckiest things for the fortunes of the drug industry is that, besides having hearts and being depressed, we all have bones and joints. When these fail us, they become a perfect target for more bad drug rip offs. The pharmaceutical industry has reached 750 billion dollars a year in sales and is poised on the cusp of hitting one trillion dollars in the next few years. 40% of that amount is spent for drugs to treat arthritis and more recently osteoporosis.

The drug companies have realized that there is significant money to be made in the bone density market. To try to decipher the complex statistical machinations that the clinical trials on biphosphonates, with trade names of Fosamax or Boniva, requires more patience, perseverance and intellect than I have. The data in these trials are divided into innumerable sub-groups so as to parse out the limited positive findings from the negative. So we have to deal with, post menopausal women with low bone density, subjects with preexisting vertebral fractures, men with hemorrhoids and on and on. The simple bottom line is that these drugs do not reduce fracture risk in the overall user population. They do reduce the risk of vertebral compression in women with low bone densities that have had a previous vertebral compression. They don't bother to tell you that vertebral compressions comprise less than 10% of total fractures and of those, 80% are asymptomatic. The over all fracture rate is not decreased and in particular, the rate of hip fracture, which has a mortality in the elderly of 30%, is not decreased.

This is all too much for me, so I decided to provide my own simplified statistical analysis. One that I can understand. Using their own data, I find the following to be true:
1. Treatment with Fosamax for one year increases bone density by 1%.
2. In head to head trials, Boniva and Fosamax are equal.
3. The overall fracture rate of patients on Fosamax treatment is 3% per year. No risk reduction is seen for non spinal and hip fractures.

Surprisingly, the overall risk of fracture in women over 65 years of age, in multiple large studies, under no treatment is 1.25% per year. **Therefore according to my statistics these drugs increase fracture rates.**

Moreover, many studies have demonstrated that the appropriate form of vitamin D and calcium supplementation reduces fracture rate , prevents bone loss and increases bone density by 1% per year.

Fosamax has been shown to prevent or delay bone healing when a fracture does occur. Bone deposition when using Fosamax is on the surface not in the trabecular matrix of the bone which in the long term will make bones more brittle- there have more than 300 reports of non traumatic femoral fractures associated with the use of Fosamax. Another major side effect of this class of drug is incapacitating bone and joint pain according to an FDA alert of January 7, 2008. Many of these cases showed slow or incomplete resolution following discontinuation of biphosphonate treatment.

A serious side effect of Fosamax is osteonecrosis of the mandible (jaw bone). By 2007, 104 law suits had been filed against Merck for this problem. A study just published in the Journal of the American Dental Association revealed an astonishing 4% of patients on an oral biphosphonate (Fosamax) suffered from osteonecrosis of the jaw even after only short-term use. Other side effects include nausea, heart burn, diarrhea, muscle cramps, ulceration of the esophagus, chest pain and blood clotting disorders.

Since one of the side effects of biphosphonates is esophageal inflammation or heart- burn, the expected drug cascade follows - that is- taking another pill for the side effects of the first pill. In this case it would be one of the heart-burn drugs such as prevacid or prilosec which, not surprisingly, within a year will increase fracture risk by more than 50%. If one of these heartburn drugs is taken for longer periods the risk of fracture increases to a whopping 250%. Apparently blocking the production of acid in the stomach prevents the

112

absorption of calcium so necessary for bone health. While we are on the subject it should be noted that taking antidepressant drugs (SSRI's) causes a 50% increase risk of fracture. Apparently not taking prozac is more effective in preventing fractures than taking Fosamax.

Looking at further data from the drug company literature filled with impressive charts to show that Boniva is as effective as Fosamax the following statement is seen: "in the overall bone fracture population **the effect of Boniva on non- vertebral fractures was similar to that of placebo"**. If that quote doesn't sum it all up, I don't know what does. We are asked to accept a plethora of side effects for a drug that exhibits no benefit beyond what a simple supplement of vitamin D and calcium in proper form would do. (A form of which was obviously avoided since all subjects in their trials were given calcium and vitamin D).
(CHOLECALCIFERAL SUPPLEMENTATION CONTROLLED TRIAL BMJ 2003.)

At this point I have to bring up the fact that as I research various drugs I am not specifically cherry picking for drugs that don't work, but I am surveying a cross section of top selling and most popular drugs. It comes as a surprise to me as well as it might to you that each time I look at another drug I find the same lack of benefit and excess toxicity. For this reason before we move on to the next topic of this chapter - arthritis - lets pause and reflect on what we have seen up to now and what it might contribute to an understanding of the chapters to follow.

We have seen incontrovertible data that many well accepted hypotheses underlying widely used drugs are not scientifically sound, and the drugs themselves are often both toxic and clinically insignificant. It is therefore obvious that the following statements are true:
It is simply crazy to not only risk death, but to actually die, from the use of a drug of marginal effectiveness and never life saving.

Doctors and drug companies always downplay or deny side effects and always exaggerate effectiveness.

If there is one certainty here, it is that the entire medical industry cannot be trusted to tell us the truth, much less be trusted with our lives and the lives of our children.

Doctors increasingly fail to understand that the destruction of immune function by drugs opens the door to infection, tumors and death and is unacceptable in exchange for temporary symptomatic relief.

You may think that I am being too hard on doctors, but I can assure you by the time you finish the final chapter of this book you will conclude that my censure has been justified and temperate. When you get angry, then you will know that you have seen the truth.

There is clearly something perverse in the human mind which allows us to ignore the obvious in favor of a belief system imposed by an authoritarian source. When that source has an agenda that is primarily money and marketing, then we are all at risk.

Imagine for a moment, that you have lived your entire live of an isolated tribal village with no contact with the outside world. Everyone in your village believes, without question, in the knowledge and wisdom of the witch doctor that treats illness with witchcraft and incantation. Now imagine that a stranger enters your village from the outside world and proceeds to tell you that the witch doctor's cures are nothing but useless superstition. Imagine what your response to this would be and calculate the chances that this stranger would leave your village alive.

Now expand in your mind your tribal world to encompass the entire earth and you will see the world we are living in today - an authoritarian and pseudo scientific illusion of reality that denies the obvious and brooks no criticism. Perhaps the best comment I can find to explain the unexplainable is to be found in a short conversation between Alice in Wonderland and the Cat:

"But I don't want to go among mad people," Alice remarked". "Oh, you can't help that" said the Cat: "we are all mad here. I'm mad. You're mad".
"How do you know I'm mad?" said Alice.
"You must be," said the Cat, "or you wouldn't have come here."----

So with this lucid explanation in mind, let's look at the new miracle treatments for the biggest money maker of them all- arthritis.

Nearly half of all Americans suffer from at least one chronic disease - 20 million more this year than had been anticipated. Researchers warn that by the year 2020, the total will exceed 160 million. Despite this ominous warning the medical industry continues to concentrate their efforts on immuno-suppressant drugs that only treat symptoms rather than ways to strengthen immune function--a course that would be preventative as well as therapeutic. This is particularly true in the efforts to treat rheumatoid arthritis and other autoimmune disorders.

The treatment of arthritis in its many forms can be divided into five primary categories:

1. Non steroidal anti-inflammatory drugs (NSAID's). These include drugs such as Ibuprofen and Naproxen as well as the cox2 inhibitors Vioxx and Celebrex.

2. Disease modifying anti rheumatic drugs (DMARDs) these are immuno-suppressive drugs such as methotrexate and cyclosporine.

3. Cortico- steroids such as prednisone.

4. Tumor necrosis factor (TNF) blockers such as Humira and Remicade.

5. Analgesics and narcotics such as acetaminophen, codeine and oxycodone.

In total, there are literally thousands of anti- arthritic medications costing consumers over 200 billion dollars a year, world wide. What are we really getting for our money and what price are we paying in toxicity and death?
First let's take a brief look at the NSAID's. There are two classes of non- steroidal anti -inflammatory drugs: cox1 inhibitors and cox2 inhibitors. There are dozens of cox1 inhibitors including aspirin, ibuprofen (Advil, Motrin) naproxen (Aleve), indomethacin (Indocin) and many more. The cox2 inhibitors, better known as: Vioxx, celebrex, Bextra and Prexige, we have met before. These latter drugs have exhibited severe heart and liver related toxicity and, with the exception of Celebrex, have been withdrawn from the market. **In multiple clinical trials this class of drug has not been shown to be superior to cox1 inhibitors in relieving arthritis pain.** It should be evident that cox2 inhibitors no longer have a place in the treatment of arthritis. But, what can be said about cox1 inhibitors? The consensus of studies shows that these drugs are neither safe nor significantly effective.

The recommendation of the American College of Rheumatology (ACR) is that analgesics such as acetominephen (Tylenol) be used preferentially as initial arthritis therapy. The ACR stated "we found no good evidence that NSAID's are superior to simple analgesics such as acetominephen, or that any one of the many NSAIDS, is more effective than the others in relieving the pain of osteoarthritis." This analysis included Celebrex. They found pain reduction with all NSAIDS only modest, that is, 10% over placebo. **In conclusion they stated "acetominephen is**

116

the drug of choice for the initial treatment of osteoarthritis pain - regardless of the severity of joint pain or the presence of clinical signs of joint inflammation".

A meta-analysis of NSAID's in placebo controlled trials published in the BMJ 2005 concluded "NSAID's can reduce short term pain in osteoarthritis slightly better than placebo, but the current analysis does not support the long term use of NSAID's for this condition, as serious adverse effects are associated with oral NSAID's."
All NSAID's have side effects including upset stomach, nausea, vomiting, heartburn, headaches, diarrhea and fatigue. More serious adverse reactions are stomach ulcers with perforation and bleeding, responsible for 25 thousand US deaths per year.

In a 2007 trial (TARGET) high risk patients had nine times the risk of heart attack and stroke when taking Ibuprofen and aspirin compared to the cox2 inhibitor Celebrex. The patients on Celebrex, in turn, had a higher risk than patients on Naproxen (Aleve). In addition, participants on Ibuprofen demonstrated significantly higher risk for congestive heart failure.
It is clear that the appropriate treatment for arthritis is analgesics such as Tylenol. Failure of control, in my opinion, should logically be treated with more potent analgesics rather than immuno-suppressive drugs which increase mortality. I fail to understand why doctors are more sanguine with the occurrence of infection, cancer and death concomitant with the use of DMARDS and TNF blockers, than they are with the possible addiction problems concomitant with the use of more effective analgesics such as codeine or oxycodone. I find the concept that immuno-suppressive drugs can be "disease modifying" preposterous. If one were to conduct a blinded clinical trial comparing oxycodone, head to head, against any arthritis treatment in use today, I can guarantee which would be more effective and less toxic by a factor of ten.

The next category of agents for treatment of rheumatoid arthritis include steroids (prednisone), DMARDS (methotrexate)and tumor necrosis factor inhibitors (Humira, Remicade) all of these modalities are immuno- suppressive and hazardous. Steroids are unacceptable for long term use due to their well known toxicity. DMARDS are also immuno suppressive and show poor efficacy despite considerable support for their long term use. The most popular of the DMARDS- methotrexate- has been reduced now to an adjuvant treatment and a base line placebo for the highly touted TNF clinical trials.

Looking at the adverse effects of the TNF blockers we find innumerable serious adverse events secondary to immuno-suppression. A Mayo clinic study in 2006 found that rheumatoid arthritis patients on TNF blockers were 3 times as likely to develop cancer or serious infections such as; pneumonia, tuberculosis or systemic fungal infection. As of September 2008 the FDA reported 45 deaths from fungal disease while taking Humira or Remicade. Clinical trials in 2004 revealed a high incidence of allergic reaction and aplastic anemia. Post marketing reports include congestive heart failure, lupus, lymphoma, blood disorders, herpes and psoriasis. All of this is perfectly predictable from a drug which suppresses immune function. In June 2008 the FDA announced a probe into increased risk of lymphoma and leukemia in children.

Lesser side effects such as stomach pain, nausea, headaches, back pain, weakness, rash, shortness of breath and dizziness are common. All of this for a mere $15,000.00 dollars per year per patient. With this in mind let's examine the purported benefits.

A metaanalysis of several trials of TNF blockers revealed the following results at 24 weeks.

Approximately 50% of subjects achieved a 20% reduction in symptoms ,compared to 20% of subjects on placebo achieving

118

a 20% reduction in symptoms. These results were achieved by imposing rigid eligibility requirements. Without these eligibility criteria the results were 20% symptomatic improvement in 20% of subjects. My mathematics suggests the following:

Since 30% of subjects (over placebo) achieved 20% improvement the **true remission rate in the overall population would be 30% x 20% or 6%.**

It is obvious that for the overall population including those not meeting the eligibility requirements the results would be less than 6% and probably less than placebo as is true for the use of Remicade in the treatment of Crohn's disease. Additionally, it is unknown whether the length of time for sustained remission extends beyond 3 months.

In the clinical trial of Remicade for treatment of Crohn's disease, an inflammatory bowel disorder, we see the same puffery and slight of hand manipulation of data.

Published in Lancet 2002 this trial was the basis for FDA approval of Remicade for treatment of Crohn's disease. The results of the primary endpoint--25% improvement at 30 weeks were shown as follows: placebo (plus single dose one time Remicade) 25%, 5mg Remicade 39%, and 10mg. Remicade 46%.

Since 50% of subjects were excluded as "non-responders" the true figures are placebo 20%, 5mg. Remicade 20% and10mg.Remicade 23%.[3% over placebo!]

At the higher and more toxic dose a 25% improvement in 3% of patients (over placebo) equals grand total overall remission rate of .075% or three quarters of one percent! With the 5mg. dose the remission rate was no greater than placebo. Such figures are laughable at best and criminal if one considers the toxicity profile of these drugs!

A simple analgesic approach to the treatment of rheumatoid arthritis would be far superior in light of the limited and short term benefit coupled with the serious, often fatal, adverse events of TNF blockers. Certainly one would

119

wonder why Dr. D's non-toxic drug ALPHAMIR, which shows 90%+ remission rate and can be taken for a lifetime, WITHOUT TOXICITY, is not available to the many sufferers of rheumatoid arthritis and other autoimmune disorders. But then, we don't have much to say about what drugs the pharmaceutical companies offer to us, or don't offer to us, as the case may be. So-- let's take a look at some of their top offerings in the next few chapters

CHAPTER XIV

THE WATER WORKS-- OR TO PEE OR NOT TO PEE (SHAKESPEER)

One of the cleverest commercials we see on TV today shows people, horses and dogs made of copper piping. Clever commercials like these are calculated to convince us that there is a wonderful and easy remedy for that "overactive bladder" that is disrupting our lives. We are told that "it's time to take control of your overactive bladder". The clear implication is that Vesicare (solifenacin) is the solution to the problem of sudden bladder urgency and frequent trips to the bathroom.

In the VENUS study, at the end of 12 weeks the primary end point was mean change in number of urgency episodes per 24 hours. The result was that **the average decrease in bathroom trips to urinate was 1 per 24 hour period.** Also, patients reporting some improvement in the degree of urgency was- 42% for Vesicare versus- 33% for placebo. [Is it possible to subjectively measure a decrease in degree of urgency of 9 % over placebo?]

In payment for 1 less trip to the bathroom per day, 27% suffered dry mouth, 15% constipation, 5% blurred vision, 5% dyspepsia, 3% fatigue, 2% dizziness and the overall rate of serious adverse events was 2%. It is doubtful that anybody who viewed the cute copper piping commercial would have suspected that they would have to exchange all these serious side effects for one less trip to the urinal per day.

While we are on the subject, we should mention another treatment for over active bladder and urinary urgency -Detrol (tolperodine). In a placebo controlled study of 1015 patients, the patients on Detrol achieved a **decrease of 0.6 urinary episodes per day or less than 1, in exchange for a side effect incidence exceeding 40%.** This should be enough said about overactive bladder.

A large percentage in men over 50 suffer from benign prostatic hypertrophy (BPH) with difficulty urinating. They are always prescribed medication by their urologists to alleviate this problem, presumably on the basis of TV commercials because apparently nobody looks at the clinical trial data.

In one TV commercial the actor hoists a huge symbolic sphere in his right hand, considerably larger than a grapefruit (presumably representing the world's largest prostate). In his left hand he then brings up a diminutive golf ball size sphere as we are informed that Avodart is the only medicine proven to shrink the prostate. This symbolic hyperbole, not withstanding, it would be appropriate to ask your urologist what he thinks of the data provided by the manufacturer of Avodart to the FDA - which is as follows:

In 3 clinical trials after, 4 years of therapy, Avodart reduced prostate volume by 24%. In addition, over 4 years Avodart reduced symptoms on a scale of 0 to 35 (with a mean baseline of 17) by 1.3 units or in other words, a symptomatic improvement of 7.7%.

Maximum urine flow rate was increased by 1 ml per second from a base line of 10 ml per second or, in other words, an increase of 10%.

In return for this miniscule and clinically unrecognizable effect, Avodart users had to suffer the following: erectile dysfunction 5%, decreased libido 3%, breast enlargement 1%, weight gain 1%, and depression 1%. How many men would be eager to get 1cc per second increase in maximum urine flow in exchange for a 5% risk of erectile dysfunction? I think the answer to this question is obvious - to everyone but urologists.

Obviously Avodart is a long term project requiring at least 2 years to reach its primary end point. However, now we find that the television ad is telling us that Flomax can alleviate our symptoms in only 1 week. Changing us from a wretched creature chained to the bathroom into a happy adventuresome elderly male now participating in a host of outings with his buddies, and no longer a prisoner of his prostate. But what is the reality?

Flomax (tamsulosin) was given in a randomized controlled trial to patients with symptomatic BPH for 12 weeks. (British Journal of Urology) The results were as follows:

There was an increase in maximum urinary flow rate (Q-MAX) in patients on Flomax compared to placebo of 1 cc. per second or 9%.

There was a decrease in total symptom score of 1.2 points or 11 %.(again, a clinically meaningless degree of improvement) The side effects of Flomax were as follows: runny or stuffy nose 18%, infection (cold/flu) 10%, back pain 8%, sore throat 6%, diarrhea 6%, dizziness 17%, abnormal ejaculation 18%.

Side effects between 1 and 5% were depression, weakness, insomnia, cough, chest pain, nausea, blurred vision and decreased libido.

I would certainly like to query my urologist if he believes the benefit of Flomax is worth the risk of the side effects I just outlined.

Again we are privy to a widely used group of drugs prescribed for millions of people who are totally unaware of the miniscule benefit they offer or of the potential risks and side effects that they create. I doubt that many would bother to pay the high price of these drugs had they been provided with this information by their urologist.

By now you should be wondering just how close to useless a drug can get and still gain FDA approval. Perhaps you have also noticed that while data presented to the FDA, may show a clinically insignificant increase in efficacy over placebo, later meta-analyses and unpublished results almost always wipe out the tiny advantage required by the FDA. The FDA does not, however, withdraw its approval when the drug is found useless, toxic or both.

A short time ago, as I have suggested that you do, I went to speak with my urologist who we will call Dr. Blank. I had been prescribed Flomax for my enlarged prostate and difficulty urinating, one month before. I was sitting in a small cubicle within his office reading a thoughtfully provided copy of modern baby care magazine when Dr. Blank rushed into the roomette - he seemed in a hurry - "how are you doing on the Flomax?" "Great" I replied "my maximum flow rate has increased from 15 to 16 cc per second! Of course, I had to buy a $10,000 piece of equipment to measure the increase but I am quite pleased with the result. Unfortunately though, I have been too dizzy to use the equipment lately - that wouldn't be because of the medicine?" I asked. Seeming not to hear the question Dr. Blank asked "how are you doing symptomatically?" "Great" I replied, "I am, symptomatically, at least 9.5% better than last month. Of course, I haven't had an orgasm this month but, that is not particularly a problem because my libido is so much lower - you don't think that it could be this medicine do you, Doc?" Dr. Blank gave me a blank stare, as if thinking, and said while exiting the room, maybe you better double up on the Flomax and I will see you again in a month".

Let's now look at a few more drugs and see if we can find a pattern. Keep in mind that I have not picked these drugs because of poor results, but primarily based on a large scale popularity and TV adds suggesting that these drugs are the best that the industry has to offer. You might recall from a previous chapter, that Eli Lilly's drug Cymbalta (an SNRI), was a failed treatment for generalized anxiety disorder (GAD) due to toxicity and lack of efficacy. Eli Lilly, however, did not give up on Cymbalta. In October 2006 Eli Lilly issued a press release saying that they had done clinical trials which found that Cymbalta significantly reduced pain in women with fibromyalgia.

The results of the studies were as follows: for men there was no difference compared to placebo. For women there was a "significant" reduction in pain compared to placebo in the first month. However, this tapered off and there was **no**

significant difference between the two groups at the end of the 12 week study.

With this result the food and drug administration regulators approved the drug for treatment of fibromyalgia in June 2008. The adverse effects of Cymbalta are as follows: nausea 35%, somnolence, insomnia and dizziness were reported between 10 and 20%, dry mouth 23%, headaches 20%. 23 other side effects some fatal, have been listed as well as severe side effects from "withdrawal syndrome" and in 18 to 24 year olds there is a 5 fold increase in suicidality. So much for the protection afforded to us by the FDA.

Another drug, Zelnorm (Tegaserod), proffered for the treatment of irritable bowl syndrome with constipation (IBS-C) was suspended and recalled by the FDA and Novartis the manufacturer, in 2007 when clinical trials showed a 1200% increase in life threatening cardiovascular events (heart attack and stroke). The FDA told Novartis it would consider allowing a limited reintroduction of Zelnorm "if a population of patients could be identified in whom the benefits of the drug outweigh the risk". In 2008 the FDA again approved Zelnorm for use in irritable bowel syndrome in women younger than 55.

We have seen what the risks are, so what are the benefits? For IBS-C, a non fatal condition consisting of abdominal pain, bloating and constipation the results in three clinical trials were as follows:

At month three the proportion of patients reporting some level of relief was 11%, 5% and 5% in the three clinical trials for a combined 7% "some" relief response over placebo. No difference was seen in trials of treated men versus placebo.

In regard to constipation, 10% of patients over placebo reported one additional bowel movement per week; however, this effect disappeared at 12 weeks. [Is this one tenth of a

126

bowel movement per week per patient? or one B.M. per patient in 10 weeks? Wow! Great! --- Rats! Gone at 12 weeks--- we knew it couldn't last.] .

Non- fatal side effects in the participants included abdominal pain, nausea, flatulence, headaches, dizziness, joint pain, vomiting and increased abdominal surgery. Post marketing reports linked Zelnorm to ischemic colitis (gangrenous bowel), cholecystitis and serious allergic reactions.

I will let you be the judge in regards to the now rather infamous "risk/benefit ratio" of this drug.

Eli Lilly in a quick move to pick up the fibromyalgia market (following the failure of Cymbalta in 2006) now put forward Lyrica (Pregabalin) at the American College of Rheumatology meeting of November 2007.

Eli Lilly reported that a placebo controlled trial of Lyrica effectively relieved pain associated with fibromyalgia.

Following a placebo run in phase (?) subjects were assigned to treatment or placebo group. Over the entire treatment period the mean difference from placebo was minus 0.38 (300 mg. dose) change from a base line mean pain score of 6.7. This amount to a whopping 5.7% reported pain decrease!

37% of subjects reported dizziness and 18% reported somnolence in using Lyrica.

Once more I suggest you use your own judgment as to the risk- benefit ratio of Lyrica as, obviously, no one else seems capable of doing it.

You might ask at this point if any of the new wonder drugs that we're shelling out billions for are of benefit. (Dare we expect such a thing?) So, let's look at a few more that we all know.

CHAPTER XV
THE GOOD, THE BAD, AND THE UGLY

Since you have gotten this far in this book - I know what you must be thinking. Allow me, as I write this chapter, to tell you what I am thinking. I am thinking that there is no literary agent that will have the fortitude to represent me in the publication of this book. If there is such an agent - no publisher will publish such a book. If there is such a publisher- no one will want to read a book about such a shocking and depressing reality. If, per chance, someone were to read this book- by the time they reach this chapter they will be thinking that this is just too much to swallow and it can't be the real story. After all, this person is telling us that we can't trust our doctor, no matter how voluminous his credentials or how pristine his white coat. Why should we believe him?

Never-the-less, I will persevere in this chapter outlining a spectrum of drugs that constitute the billion dollar club in an effort to pry open your minds a little further. If we succeed in that we will then be able to proceed into the final chapters which make the facts in the first fifteen look like minor peccadilloes.

To set the stage I would like to share with you a conversation between with friend Walter:

Walter and I have been close friends for many years and we share lunch each week during which I harangue poor Walter about the latest revelation of medical chicanery that was leaving me both angry and incredulous. This particular week the topic over our shared marinated beef brochette happened to be statin drugs. For once Walter expressed some interest. "My doctor has me on Crestor", he said. With that I pulled out a copy of my chapter "Enter Lipitor" and also a file two inches thick of clinical studies on the cholesterol myth and statin drugs. I shoved them into his hands and said "you show these to your doctor and see what he has to say--But first I want to tell you a little story--

George Washington came down with a fever and upper respiratory illness on a certain Friday night. His physician came in and bled him that night taking 12 ounces of blood, but

129

without improvement. The next day he was again bled copiously twice more, but still without improvement. So another 32 ounces of blood was taken. By Saturday night he was dead."

After a moment of reflection Walter asked "and your point is"? "Well", I said, "if it took 2500 years for doctors to realize that bleeding was a bad therapy, how can you trust them to realize that they are mistaken now?"

Two days later Walter called me to report on what the doctor told him. "Oh, we discuss these things all the time at meetings- and if we were wrong about this we would certainly know it." (This sounds to me a lot like "are you going to trust me - or are your going to trust your lying eyes.")

"So are you satisfied with that response," I asked. "No, said Walter "not really." "Then are you going to stop the Crestor?" I queried. "Well" he said, "I am taking the lowest possible dose."   "Didn't you read the studies I gave you?" I asked. "Yes", he said "but it's a bad idea to get my cardiologist mad at me."

I'll leave it at that - if I can't convince my friend Walter to abandon "mindless trust" what chance is there for a universal epiphany?

With that said, we must do some further spade work before moving on to an abyss from which there may be no return.

Surely, if we are to find a drug which breaks the pattern and we can agree that it is a good drug - meaning effective and non toxic - it should be among the worlds most prescribed. The top 20 sellers are all three billion dollar or more blockbusters. Let's start with number one, Lipitor at 15 billion dollars earnings.

If you are still thinking that you would like to take a statin drug I suggest that you reread the chapters on cholesterol and Lipitor - this time with your eyes open. No statin drug shows any mortality benefit. They are all unacceptably toxic and the data are overwhelming that lower cholesterol levels increase mortality in every group or cohort studied. Lipitor and all statins get an unequivocally bad drug rating.

Number 3 and 4, Nexium and Prevacid come in at 9 billion dollars, both are proton pump inhibitors. They prevent the production of acid in the stomach and are effective in the treatment of heart-burn and ulcers. These drugs are not intended or recommended for use for more than 6 weeks. Common side effects seen in more that 5% of users include headache, diarrhea and stomach pain. The list of side effects in clinical trials and post marketing reports exceed a hundred and fifty including fatal cases of toxic epidermal necrolysis. With this side effect profile it would be wise to adopt an alternate approach to heartburn relief. Lastly, long term use (4-7 years) of Nexium leads to a 3-5 times increased risk of hip fracture which has 30% mortality in the elderly. Proton pump inhibitors like Nexium prevent production of acid which in turn prevents the absorption of calcium.

An interesting fact is that Prilosec is essentially identical to Nexium and both are made by the same company Astra-Zeneca, who unleashed a media blitz to promote the "little purple pill" at seven times the cost of the identical over the counter drug Prilosec.

Next on the list is Advair (6 billion), an inhalant containing salmeterol for the treatment of chronic asthma. Salmeterol is a long acting beta agonist (LABA). Advair used for asthma results in a 6 times greater incidence of asthma related death according to a study appearing in the Annals of Internal Medicine. The research doctor had this to say, "These asthma deaths are generally in healthy adults. We estimate that approximately 4 thousand of the 5 thousand asthma deaths that occur in the US each year are actually caused by these long acting beta agonists and we urge that these agents be taken off the market." Conclusion: Advair joins the list of bad drugs.

131

The next 6 billion dollar drug we will consider is Plavix, a "blood thinner" used to prevent heart attack and stroke. In the CHARISMA study done in 2006 on 15,600 high risk patients (with clinically evident cardiovascular disease) the rate of death was almost twice in the Plavix group as in the placebo (plus ASA) group. The rate of bleeding was 3.8% in the Plavix group compared to 2.6% in the placebo plus ASA group. The Charisma data indicates that Plavix plus ASA is responsible for nearly half of post heart attack deaths with long term use.

Next on the list of top 20 drugs are a group of antipsychotics including Zoloft, Effexor, Risperdal, Seroquel and Zyperexa. The antidepressants such as Zoloft and Effexor were dealt with in a previous chapter and were shown to be both ineffective and toxic. Atypical antipsychotics as group - Seroquel, Zyprexa and Risperdal have been shown to cause serious side effects such as pancreatitis, diabetes and stroke. Thirty thousand law- suits have been filed against Zyprexa in relation to development of diabetes secondary to its use. A study published in the British Medical Journal showed that the use of Seroquel in nursing homes doubled the rate of cognitive decline and increased the death rate 2.5 times.

A more recent study in the Lancet showed that the use of atypical antipsychotics more than doubled the death rate. Numerous studies have shown that these drugs are ineffective in improving the quality of life of these patients.

Norvasc (amlodipine), an antihypertensive known as an ACE inhibitor, comes in at 3 billion dollars. The ALLHAT Study showed that a diuretic, hydrochlorthiazide, was superior to Norvasc in effectiveness with less toxicity. The cost of hydrochlorthiazide is 36 dollars per year compared to Norvasc at 724 dollars per year.

In a series of studies, babies born to women taking ACE inhibitors had a 7 to 10% incidence of serious birth defects. In an edition of the New England Journal of Medicine Dr. J M Friedman, a medical geneticist at the University of British Columbia, stated "the drug companies have known that these drugs pose a danger to the fetus and they should have been banned in pregnant women 15 years ago - this is just another blatant example of drug companies putting profits ahead of lives."

Another class of drugs in the top 20 reaching 10 billion dollars in revenue is produced by recombinant DNA technology. Epogen, Procrit and Aranesp are used to combat anemia in chemotherapy patients. A JAMA study showed a 10% increase in the risk of death in patients on these drugs as well as a more than 50% increase risk of dangerous blood clots. The FDA has issued warnings on these drugs.

The next group in the top 20 is the TNF blockers Remicade and Embrel. These were discussed at length in a previous chapter and showed both poor effectiveness and unacceptable long term toxicity.

The final candidate in the top 20 is Singulair (montelukast), an inhalant for allergies and asthma. The results of multiple trials on the use of Singulair were as follows:

With a primary endpoint of percent change of Forced expiratory volume in one second (FEV1), at 15 weeks Singulair achieved a 4% increase over placebo.

In a six week treatment period for seasonal allergy Singulair improved symptoms 6% over placebo.

In Perennial rhinitis a 6 week treatment period with Singulair improved allergic symptoms 4% over placebo.

The following adverse events occurred in 2% or more of subjects: fever, cough, abdominal pain, diarrhea, headaches, rhinorrhea, sinusitis, otitis, rash, ear pain, gastroenteritis, eczema, hives, pneumonia, dermatitis.

I will let you be the judge on this one - I'm tired of being the bad guy- but I defy anyone to be able to notice a 4 to 6% improvement in allergy symptoms.

Unfortunately the top 20 candidates didn't help us to find a good drug. But let's not give up yet. There are a number of blockbuster drugs that only recently have dropped out of the top 20 that we can look at.

How about Premarin? That's been a major drug for many years. The Women's Health Initiative, a long term federal study out of the UCLA Medical Center, showed that women on hormones (Premarin, Prempro) were twice as likely to have heart problems and breast cancer. Following this report Premarin dropped out of the top 10. The makers of Prempro, Wyeth Pharmaceuticals, paid ghost writers to produce medical journal articles favorable to Prempro and at least one of these articles was published after the federal study showing a doubling of breast cancer rates. (Quelle surprise!!).

In our quest for a good drug maybe the TV commercial favorites will provide what we don't seem to be able to find in the top 20. A rather touching commercial I saw recently portrayed a family that recovered their beloved grandfather from the oblivion of Alzheimer's and brought him back into the bosom of the family. All accomplished with the miracle drug Aricept. Is it possible that the commercial overstated its effectiveness? Well let's see what the research states about Aricept, as well as Exelon and Reminyl, all "me too" Alzheimer's drugs knows as cholinesterase inhibitors.

A British Medical Journal revue identified 22 published studies that tested the use of these 3 drugs in the treatment of Alzheimer's disease. No study found anything more than a minimal benefit with respect to any of the drugs when compared to placebo. One study showed a very slight delay in progression (No improvement) but this effect disappeared at 6 months. Could it be that the TV commercial was calculated to

134

sell drugs by a callous appeal to guilt and false hopes? (Quelle Surprise!!! Again)

Another study of Aricept in vascular dementia found Aricept no better than placebo, however; unfortunately, there were 11 deaths during the 24 week study in the Aricept group and none in the placebo group.

Another TV favorite, Claritin, is the "non drowsy" antihistamine for all our allergy woes. Even though Claritin isn't in the billion dollar class surely it will not disappoint us in our search for a good drug----- Well, I spoke too soon. It turns out that studies show that Claritin is effective in reduction of allergy symptoms by a mere 6% over placebo. This level of effectiveness, I submit, is indistinguishable from a sugar pill by any individual.

For this meager 6% improvement 12% of user's reported headache, 8% dizziness, 4% fatigue and 3% dry mouth.

Perhaps encouraged by the lack of efficacy of Claritin, another drug company recently introduced a nasal spray for allergy treatment called Omnaris (ciclesonide). Realizing that a drug doesn't require any level of effectiveness to be sold, Omnaris states in the package insert the following: "in the 12 week trial in patients with perennial allergic rhinitis, **none of the ciclesonide doses were statistically significantly different from placebo".** Maybe they figure that if Claritin can do it, they could also. One thing I am sure of though is that the doctor who gave Omnaris samples to my daughter certainly didn't read the package insert first!

I would like to mention a few words about the sleep aide Ambien (zolpidem) but, unfortunately, the list of side effects including sleep driving and sleep eating, would fill the rest of this book - all for the 30 to 40 minutes of increased sleep time reported in clinical trials.

Up to now we have been discussing drugs still marketed and being prescribed. There are however, many dozens of "uglier" drugs which have been pulled from the market, often long after the drug company knew of its lethal potential. Vioxx was one of these - Merck however, has not given up on COX 2 inhibitors and has set its sights on a new arthritis blockbuster called Arcoxin. Merck, of course, contends that Arcoxin is safer than Vioxx as they again immerse their snouts in the trough of arthritis sales.

In March of 2005, the New Zealand Health Authority issued the strongest warning so far on COX 2 inhibitors, ruling that the increased risk of cardiovascular events outweighs the benefits of these drugs. Merck chooses, however, to throw the dice one more time with a drug we simply don't need.

We must by now be exhausted by what appears to be the never ending search for the mythical good drug, so this chapter ends here. But, be forewarned, these chapters have been only a preliminary to the main events in the chapters to follow.

CHAPTER XVI
FOR THE BIRDS

As I begin writing this chapter, delving ever deeper into the sordid morass of pharmaceutical profiteering, I was struck by the twisted irony in the breaking news of the day. A prominent investor from a long line of aristocratic Frenchman was found sitting at his desk with both wrists slashed. This gentleman had placed over a billion dollars into the fifty billion dollar Ponzi scheme orchestrated by the affable and cherubic Bernard Madoff.

This death was perhaps only the first to come, among the many victims of Mr. Madoff - a consequence of doubtful concern to Bernie. Beyond doubt, few would have believed for a moment that this cherubic old man could have perpetrated such a massive fraud on the financial elite of the world. Millionaires, billionaires, bankers and sophisticated caretakers of billions, all swindled by Bernie - another unbelievable reality, but true never-the-less.

A perfect analogy as to how one person can influence" sophisticated opinion" which cascades down as an all encompassing lie, sustained by greed, ego and denial. Madoff certainly did it. Another individual named Ancel Keys started another such cascade when he rigged the data purporting to show that a high fat diet was the cause of heart disease. The Nobel Laureate Linus Pauling did it when he obsessively hawked antioxidants and vitamin C as cure- alls.

Now we again have another cascade of misinformation begun by a single individual named "Henny Penny" who's warning that the sky is falling has thrust us into a three billion dollar medical scramble to save us from the dreaded scourge of the avian flu. An epidemic falling from the sky.

According to the CDC, influenza strikes between 5 and 20% of the population each year and more than two hundred thousand people are hospitalized from flu complications and about thirty- six thousand people die.

The CDC advises flu vaccine as the first line of defense against flu and the antiviral drugs Tamiflu and Relenza as the second line of defense. As of this writing the

CDC has advised routine flu vaccines for everyone from 6 months of age and up. This essentially includes the entire population at an annual cost of ten billion dollars. Beyond this, the CDC recommends Tamiflu as a second line of defense because it is claimed to reduce the duration of influenza symptoms (if taken within the first 48 hours) by one day.

Introduced in 1999, sales of Tamiflu were understandably poor. However, following media hysteria, trumpeting the imminent pandemic of avian flu as a potential death sentence for over a hundred and fifty million people, things changed. There then began a massive program of stock-piling of Tamiflu in preparation for the arrival of the world- wide pandemic of Avian flu.

In the light of all of this, the following questions must be addressed:

1. Is the CDC telling us the truth about the dangers and death toll of influenza?
2. Is the drug Tamiflu an effective treatment for either seasonal influenza or for avian flu?
3. Is there credible evidence that the flu vaccine is effective in preventing flu, flu like illness, secondary complications, or death?

We should be well aware by now that it is a lethal mistake to uncritically accept any position taken by the CDC or advised by medical professionals. Consequently we will analyze the claim by the CDC that seasonal influenza kills thirty- six thousand people every year.

The fact is that these deaths are almost entirely due to pneumonia secondary to influenza like illness. The influenza virus accounts for only 10% of all influenza like illnesses. In addition, there are over a billion upper respiratory infections each year and a million cases of pneumonia leading to 40 thousand deaths. That being the case, the contribution of influenza to these pneumonia deaths is miniscule.

139

The conclusion that influenza is responsible for the majority of pneumonia deaths is preposterous. In actuality, according to the national center for medical statistics, death from flu rarely exceeds 1000 per year and in the year 2001 was 257. Only 10% of these deaths were in persons under 65 years of age and the majority of those were individuals suffering from other diseases or who were immuno-compromised. Therefore, the CDC's position is more aligned with pharmaceutical company's agendas then to provide valid information.

The next question: is Tamiflu an effective treatment for either seasonal influenza or avian flu? Let's see.

Published in Prescire Int. June 2003 - Tamiflu, an antiviral agent with little impact on influenza.

A review of three placebo controlled trials evaluating Tamiflu as a treatment for influenza at a dosage of 75mg twice daily:

"Tamiflu shortened duration of symptoms by about 24 hours. There was no evidence that Tamiflu prevented complications. Nausea and vomiting was more common in treated patients. The poor risk- benefit ratio argues against the use of this drug."

China Medical Journal - January 2003
A double blind placebo controlled trial of Tamiflu for treatment of influenza: The median duration of illness was 91.6 hours in the Tamiflu group and 95 hours in the placebo group. Adverse events in the treated group were rash, gastrointestinal symptoms and neurological symptoms. (Despite this meager 3.5 hour difference, the authors, not surprisingly, concluded that Tamiflu was effective and well tolerated!!)

Annals of Pharmacological Therapy - January 2001.
Neuramidase inhibitors: Zanamivir (Relenza) and Oseltamivir
(Tamiflu).
Treatment with Zanamivir or Oseltamivir reduced symptom
time by approximately 0 .7-1.5 days. Gastrointestinal adverse
effects were 10%.

When biostatistician Michael Elsahoff and FDA reviewers
examined Relenza they had this to say: "Relenza was no more
effective than placebo in treating flu symptoms among
American patients and was potentially unsafe for flu patients
with asthma or other respiratory disease.

The FDA issued advisory following reports of 22 deaths
following the use of Relenza. **Glaxo said** it was "difficult to
determine" whether Relenza caused the deaths. None of
which surprised Elsahoff who said "even if you accept the
company line, that it knocks a day off the flu, a day is not
much when you compare it to your life."

A study in asthmatic patients in 2004 demonstrated a slight
improvement (3.4%) in forced expiration volume (FEV1) but,
no earlier resolution of influenza symptoms (67 versus 71
hours).

In March 2007, Japan's Health Ministry warned that Tamiflu
should not be given to those aged 10 to 19. They cited
neurological and psychological disorders as possible adverse
effects including impaired consciousness, abnormal behavior
and hallucinations. According to Japan's Health Ministry
between 2004 and March 2007, 15 people aged 10 to 19 had
been injured or killed by jumps or falls from buildings after
taking Tamiflu and one 17 year died after he jumped in front
of a truck. An investigation of the Japanese data was
completed in 2007: it found that 128 patients had been
reported to behave abnormally after taking Tamiflu.

Health Canada's Bulletin 2006 said that since February 2000 84 Canadians had had adverse reactions after taking the drug, including 10 who died and 7 adults who reported psychiatric events. In 2008 there have been 13 reported adverse events including the deaths of 3 women.

Despite this underwhelming level of effectiveness against seasonal flu, more that 80 countries have been convinced to stock- pile millions of doses of Tamiflu as a first line defense against a potentially mutated form of Avian flu which could spread from person to person.

This mutated form, we are warned by medical authorities, could kill more than 150 million people in the world's greatest pandemic.

To this date, there have been 389 cases of Avian flu (H5N1 virus) and 245 deaths. This is a death rate of 63% despite the use of Tamiflu. A report in the New England Journal of Medicine by Dr. Menno De Jong of the Hospital for Tropical Diseases in Ho Chi Minh City, Vietnam, said that 4 of 8 recent patients treated with Tamiflu died. Dr. De Jong has treated the most cases of Avian flu in the world: 95 H5N1 patients of which 42 died. **Of those treated with Tamiflu 70% died.**

A statement by Keiji Fukuda, a scientist from the WHO's Global Influenza program commented "this is no cause for alarm. Some resistance was inevitable with any kind of drug. The findings published in the New England Journal of Medicine that 4 of 8 recent patients died despite the use of Tamiflu indicates that more research is needed into how best to use the drug."

At this point one might be permitted to wonder, in view of the total absence of efficacy, why the question of resistance is even an issue. Either way it doesn't work- and the term "resistant" becomes a euphemism for ineffective.

It should be clear to the highly placed "medical experts" recommending the stock -piling of Tamiflu that even if Tamiflu actually was effective to any degree, the rapid mutation of influenza virus would nullify such effectiveness in short order. Samples taken from 40 countries show resistant strains have reached 31% world wide and are increasing rapidly.

Without doubt, the mutations that will allow for person- to- person transmission will render such a virus 100% resistant to these drugs. Up to now all cases have been associated with close contact with infected poultry. I am quite sure that the experts recommending the stock- piling of Tamiflu know full well that it will be rendered useless for these reasons. (Presuming that a 70% death rate with Tamiflu is not useless!) In fact resistant strains have already reached 100% in South Africa and 70% in Norway. I suppose, however, that the issue of Resistance is of no real concern to them since the drug is totally ineffective anyway.

If you think that the medical elite of the world is truly concerned about the deaths of a few hundred or a few million young people from avian flu the following communications will be enlightening. I could furnish hundreds of similar responses and most don't bother to reply at all. In this case it's about flu but it could just as well be about AIDS or SARS or any pestilence that provides them a cloak of high importance. Following a recent rash of deaths in Hong Kong I sent the following letter to Dr. York Chow at the Hong Kong Ministry of Health:

Dear Professor York Chow:

Kindly allow me to introduce myself. I have served in the position of Chief Director of Research at the Kenya Medical Research Institute (KEMRI) for a number of years. We have developed a new antiviral agent which has proven highly effective in a broad spectrum of viral diseases including AIDS, Influenza and hepatitis.

ALPHAMIR has been approved by the Kenyan Pharmacy board and is without toxicity of any kind. ALPHAMIR is an immune stimulant and has a potent antitoxin effect. We have had broad experience with this modality and are of the strong opinion that it would be highly effective in the therapy of H5N1 Influenza. It is easily administered as sublingual drops and organisms cannot develop resistance.

I am attaching documentation on ALPHAMIR for your perusal and I am most anxious to forward a supply to you for use in Avian Flu patients who you may see in the near future and who now face greater than 65% mortality.

It is most unfortunate that so many young people have to die for political reasons when a simple and effective therapy is available that is totally non-toxic.

If this is of interest please contact me by phone or email at your earliest convenience.

Most respectfully,

Stephen D. Herman M.D.

I received the following reply:

Dear Dr. Herman:

Thank You very much for your letter of January 19 addressed to Dr. York Chow.

I wish to inform you that if you intend to supply your product to Hong Kong you should first obtain its registration in Hong Kong. I attach herewith the relevant guidance notes on registration of pharmaceutical products in Hong Kong.

Yours Sincerely,

Anthony Chan, Chief Pharmacist Department of Health, Hong Kong SAR.

(No mention of anyone dying--or the 150 million pandemic deaths they express so much concern about)

TO WHICH I REPLIED:

Dear Anthony Chan;

I have received your email regarding procedure for drug registration and I thank you for your prompt reply, however, with all due respect, I am astonished at the substance of your reply. Did you read the letter at all? I have no desire to put the drug on sale--I was hoping there would be a person in a position of authority who was concerned about increasing numbers of unnecessary deaths of young people from H5N1 influenza which has a 65% death rate.

In addition, under paragraph 6 part C this technology is exempt from this requirement. I am continually amazed at the political barriers erected and maintained by medical authorities who care more for their bureaucratic control measures than the lives of their people. My purpose was to provide free samples through Dr. Chow in an attempt to provide a lifesaving measure. Perhaps this is not quite understandable or this may conflict with the absurd and shabby Tamiflu agenda. I would most appreciate a more enlightening reply as to the reason such a life saving new technology is of no apparent interest.

Most Respectfully,

Stephen D. Herman M.D.
Chief Director of Research, KEMRI.

Of course, I received no reply to this letter and I never will. Medicines are a business and the shop doors are closed and barred to all but the big money people. Everyone is carefully guarding those doors and the tears for the dying are crocodilian.

The CDC reported in December 2008 that a common strain of seasonal influenza in the US this winter is 100% resistant to Tamiflu. Since influenza is responsible for only a small percentage of influenza like illness it would be totally counter productive to contemplate using Tamiflu at the onset of such an illness even if there could be slight benefit.

Put in another way, ten people would have to take Tamiflu and suffer all the adverse events and side effects, for one person to have his symptoms reduced by one day. If that

145

one person happened to have the strain that was 100% resistant--well, I guess we would even lose that one day.

If all this sounds more than ridiculous than you are seeing what I am seeing with clarity--none of this passes the smell test, much less rigorous scientific validation.

If Avian flu is of such monumental concern to health authorities one wonders why they would stock- pile a drug proven to be useless in the treatment of Avian flu and at the same time so carefully ignore a proven and effective antiviral agent as Dr. D's Alphamir. Alphamir is not only strikingly effective in influenza, as well as the entire spectrum of viral URI's, but in addition, viruses cannot develop resistance to Alphamir.

In fact, Alphamir stands out as the only real defense possibility against avian flu and the AID's virus as well. Since this is of no apparent interest to the" medical experts' what is their real concern? A hundred and fifty million deaths or the loss of the huge cash flow from vaccines and drugs that they know don't work and won't work.

THE INFLUENZA VACCINE

Should we all get a flu shot as the CDC recommends and a surfeit of media hype proclaims? Or are we looking at another 10 billion dollar pharmaceutical swindle? Let's look at the data:

Archives of Pediatric and Adolescent Medicine October 2008:

A study looking at influenza vaccination of UK children has found no benefits for hospitalization or doctor visits. Vaccine effectiveness in this study was as low as 7%. Commenting on this study Dr. Peter Szilagyl, a pediatrician at the Strong Memorial Hospital in Rochester New York stated "significant influenza vaccine effectiveness could not be demonstrated for any season, age or setting."

146

Another very recent study which examined data from a 2003 Canadian Health Survey of more than 134 thousand people found patients with asthma vaccinated against influenza were 80% more likely to experience exacerbations than unvaccinated controls.

When Dr. Tom Jefferson led the team of researchers and reviewers (2005) at the Cochrane Vaccines field on an exhaustive review of the world medical literature, they scrutinized all the studies that had been done on influenza vaccination and found that the benefits were "wildly over estimated". They found that flu vaccines have little or no effect on things such as hospital stay, time off work, or even death resulting from influenza and its complications - especially in elderly people.

INFLUENZA VACCINATION; POLICY VERSUS EVIDENCE, Dr. Jefferson's follow up report encapsulating the teams findings was published in the British Medical Journal- October 2006. Looking at the push to vaccinate all babies with influenza vaccine starting at 6 months of age, Dr. Jefferson's team reviewed the existing literature on flu vaccination of children and said "in children under 2 years, inactivated vaccine had the same field efficacy as placebo."

Researchers from the National Institute of Allergy and Infections Diseases (NIAID) found no correlation between an increase in flu vaccine coverage over the past 2 decades and a decrease in influenza-related deaths among the elderly.
    The percentage of elderly Americans who got annual flu shots rose steadily from around 15% before 1980 to 65% in 2001. The dramatic increase in coverage should have led to a dramatic drop in flu death. "This is not what we found," said researcher, Lone Simonsen, PhD.

A Canadian study from the University of Alberta published in the September 2008 issue of the American Journal of

Respiratory and Critical Care calls into question previous studies that found a substantial benefit from influenza vaccine. They found a "healthy-user" effect that confounded test results. In fact, it's most likely that factors that are likely to decrease chances of having been vaccinated - low socioeconomic status and frailty - also contributed to poor natural immunity and it's the latter that is the main reason for flu deaths- not lack of vaccination.

A September 25, 2008 study from the US found that influenza vaccination may save many fewer older patients lives than generally claimed. Commenting on this study Dr. Tom Jefferson and his colleagues Carlo Di Pietrantoni, PhD. Both of the Cochrane vaccine field said these cherished vaccination policies may need to be revisited. "We must never again allow layers of poor research to mask substantial uncertainty about the effects of a public- health intervention and present a falsely optimistic view of policy."

In Canada, Flu Watch is a public health program which gathers and reports on the relative incidence of influenza cases throughout the year. Laboratory testing year in and year out shows that the majority of influenza illnesses are not associated with the influenza virus, but arise from other pathogens unaffected by the vaccine. On average, the influenza virus is associated with only 10% of people presenting with flu- like illnesses.

When one considers that vaccines are often 30 to 70% mismatched with the season's virus strains and that only 10% of influenza like illnesses are true influenza. Thus the theoretical maximum possibility (but not the minimum possibility) of effectiveness of the vaccine is often less then 10% and sometimes as low as 3%. In 2008 the CDC announced that the flu vaccine didn't match the B strain and stated two of the three vaccine components were off target.

In 2006 an independent analysis by the internationally renowned Cochrane collaboration of world wide influenza vaccine studies, published in the British Medical Journal, concluded there is little scientific proof that inactivated influenza vaccine is safe and effective for children and adults. Cochrane reviews are considered the gold standard for determining the effectiveness of health care intervention.

The 15 member advisory committee of the CDC now recommends influenza vaccination covering 84% of the US population or 256 million Americans at a cost of 10 billion dollars. Almost all the ACIP members who make these recommendations have financial ties to the vaccine industry.
The CDC mounts a well orchestrated campaign each season to generate interest and demand for flu shots. Along with posters for the public, flyers and health care provider material, it encourages doctors to urge flu shots.
Medical groups, non medical organizations and the media trumpet CDC released messages on influenza, warning that flu kills 36 thousand per year and that flu vaccine is the best defense against flu.

An article by the Group Health Center for Health Studies in Seattle to determine if flu vaccines are effective in protecting older people against developing pneumonia was published in the Lancet in 2008.
 The Group Health Study found that flu shots do not protect elderly people against developing pneumonia. Pneumonia occurs with equal frequency in people over age 65 with or without a flu shot.   As one vaccine researcher puts it "I think the evidence base for mortality benefits from flu shots we have leaned on is not valid" -

Lancet Infectious Disease 2007.
There is also a lack of evidence that young children benefit from flu shots. A systematic review of 51 studies involving 260 thousand children age 6 to 23 months found no evidence

149

that the flu vaccine is any more effective than a placebo - Cochrane Data Base System Review 2006.

Randomized controlled trials are the most reliable way to determine the efficacy and safety of a given treatment. No randomized trial shows that flu shots reduce mortality from influenza or flu related pneumonia. The absolute risk of contracting influenza is reduced by flu vaccine by a meager 1%.

Three serious and acknowledged adverse reactions to the flu vaccine are arthritis, anaphylactic shock and Guillain - Barre Syndrome. (And Alzheimer's disease)

Further comments by the Cochrane Report are as follows:

"The findings are sobering; there is a gap between evidence and public policy. The optimism and confidence of some predictions of viral circulation and of the impact of inactivated vaccines, which are at odds with the evidence, is striking. Evidence from systematic reviews show that inactivated vaccines have little or no effect on the effect measured. Little comparative evidence exists on the safety of these vaccines. There is no evidence to support the number of deaths attributed to the flu by the CDC.

Our public health policies are not even remotely evidence-based. Rather, our public health policies are faith-based decrees by government authorities - no better than voodoo medicine.

The CDC appears to be acting on behalf of flu vaccine manufacturers - even as the evidence shows the vaccine to be worthless at best."

A study published in Vaccine 2006 - Incidence of Influenza in Ontario following the Universal Influenza Immunization Campaign:

The purpose of this study from the University of Ottawa was to determine whether the incidence of influenza in Ontario,

Canada has decreased following the introduction of the Universal Influenza immunization campaign in 2000[UIIC]. All laboratory confirmed influenza cases in Ontario, from Jan. 1990 to Aug. 2005 were analyzed. They found that there has not been a decrease in the mean monthly influenza rate following the introduction of the UIIC. Despite increased vaccine distribution and major financial resources expended toward promotion, the incidence of influenza in Ontario has not decreased.

In an editorial in Infectious News Lone Simonen et al. stated the following, "we could not find the expected decline in adjusted influenza related mortality from 1980 to 2001 despite an increase in vaccine coverage of the elderly from about 15% to about 65%.

Epidemiologists in the United Kingdom recently demonstrated and corrected for self selection bias in their cohort's study, by comparing vaccine effectiveness estimates during the influenza season to vaccine effectiveness in the peri-influenza period just outside the influenza season when no vaccine effect could reasonably be expected. They reported that vaccinated elderly were 20% less likely than unvaccinated elderly to die from any cause during influenza periods - and also 20% less likely to die in Peri-influenza period. **They therefore correctly adjusted their vaccine effectiveness estimate to be zero percent in terms of prevention of all cause mortality.**

INFLUENZA IN JAPAN

A mass influenza vaccination program for school age children was started in 1960, and about 3 million children were vaccinated. In 1976 the compulsory system was introduced and 17 million children were vaccinated. This program was unique in the world and the government believed it would avoid the influenza epidemic. This was a wrong hypothesis.

Since the 80's vaccination use was constant at about 60% per year, but the incidence rate per 100 thousand of influenza went from 5 to 60 despite the vaccination rate. Since 1989 vaccination use decreased rapidly to 20%, but there was no increase in the influenza rate.
Influenza incidence rates between vaccinated and non vaccinated cities in Japan.

City A Vaccination uptake below 1% - influenza incidence 43%.

City B Vaccination uptake 90% - influenza incidence 40%.

City C Vaccination uptake 77% - influenza incidence 43%.

City D Vaccination uptake 76% - influenza incidence 52%.

A similar study was documented in 1985 with similar results. It was recommended that influenza programs be ceased.

Adverse reactions to influenza in Japanese vaccination program.

A mass study of adverse events secondary to the Influenza vaccine was conducted in 1987 involving about 400 thousand children.
The total adverse reaction rate was 254 per million. From 1972 to 1979 the total number of deaths was 50. Cases of severe developmental retardation numbered 65 and intractable epilepsy numbered 35.

INFLUENZA VACCINE AND PREGNANCY

From the Journal of American Physicians and Surgeons 2006. Influenza Vaccine and Pregnancy:

A critical assessment of the recommendation of the advisory committee on immunization practices (ACIP) by David M. Ayoub, MD. And F. Edward Yazbak, MD.

Influenza vaccination during all trimesters of pregnancy is now universally recommended in the United States. We critically reviewed the influenza vaccination policy of the CDC advisory committee and the citations that were used to support their recommendation.

The ACIP's citations and the current literature indicate that influenza infection is rarely a threat to a normal pregnancy, however; there is no convincing evidence of the effectiveness of influenza vaccination during this critical period. No studies have adequately accessed the risk of influenza vaccination during pregnancy, and animal safety testing is lacking.

Thimerosal, a mercury based preservative present in most inactivated formulations of the vaccine have been implicated in human neurodevelopment disorders, including autism, and a broad range of animal and experimental reproductive toxicities including teratogenicity, mutagenicity, and fetal death. Thimerosal is classified as a human teratogen.

The ACIP policy recommendation of routinely administering the influenza vaccine during pregnancy is ill advised and unsupported by current scientific literature, and it should be withdrawn. Use of Thimerosal during pregnancy should be contraindicated.

It should be noted that Holmes et al. determined that **mothers of autistic children received 6 times more Thimerosal-preserved RHO D immuno-globulin than mothers of neurotypical children,** strongly implying a role of prenatal mercury exposure in adverse developmental outcome.

A large study by Black and his associates at the Kaiser Permanente HMO was undertaken to assess the impact of

153

influenza during pregnancy. There was no statistical difference in illness rates among the vaccinated and unvaccinated women or their offspring.

Munoz et al. also failed to demonstrate effectiveness of influenza vaccination in pregnancy during 5 influenza seasons. Rates of acute upper respiratory tract infection did not significantly differ between vaccinated and unvaccinated women. **Paradoxically, the authors found 4 times as many ILI (influenza-like-illness) - related hospitalizations in vaccinated women,** an observation similar to that of NEUZIO et al. These observations not only challenge vaccine effectiveness, but also raise concern that vaccination actually carries an added risk of ILI. (Later proven to be true)

If the weight of these data are not convincing, I will refer you (in desperation) to the Armed Forces Health surveillance Center Department of Defense Influenza Report, November 2008.

In their report of the incidence rate of pneumonia with influenza (P&I) and influenza-like-illness (ILI) among active duty service members, US overall, influenza season 2008 - 2009, the numbers were as follows:

ILI vaccinated - 5.0 per 1000 person week
ILI unvaccinated - 3.0 per 1000 person week
P&I vaccinated - 0.4 per 1000 person week
P&I unvaccinated - 0.2 per 1000 person week

These data clearly show a **significant increase in both pneumonia associated with influenza and an increase in influenza- like- illness among the vaccinated population.**
This paradoxical effect of vaccination has been noted before in several studies.

INFLUENZA VACCINE AND ALZHEIMER'S DISEASE

154

In 1976 a "swine flu scare" impelled the U.S. government to initiate an emergency program of vaccination throughout the country. The initial target was to be 220 million persons. Special laws were passed to indemnify the vaccine manufacturers of any liability from adverse effects of the vaccine.

Over 46 million persons received the vaccine before mounting deaths from heart attacks and a host of cases of paralysis due to Guillain-Barre syndrome (GBS) surfaced following vaccine injection. The program was summarily shut down. The final result was over 300 deaths and more than 4000 cases of GBS.

Just what was the impetus for such a program pushed so hard by the CDC and pressed into action by Presidents Carter and Ford? The Ford family was shown on T.V. receiving their vaccine---President Carter refused to take his. The facts are these:

The first case of swine influenza was January 19, 1976 in a trainee recruit at Fort Dix New Jersey. This recruit was hospitalized and died of pneumonia following a strenuous 30 mile training march. A new strain of influenza was isolated, (A-New Jersey or swine flu). Subsequent to this there were 4 additional cases of pneumonia among the recruits in whom A-New Jersey was suspected. All recovered. [All recruits had received flu vaccine which could have resulted in abnormal blood titers of antibodies to A-New Jersey].

That was it-- there were no further cases after February 9 (3 weeks later)--no further hospitalizations and no further deaths. No case of suspected A-New Jersey influenza was ever seen outside of Fort Dix.

Never-the-less, a massive program with an untested vaccine was begun 8 months later in October, without a single additional case having occurred. We have seen how this exercise ended with the suspension of the program 176 million short of its targeted goal less than 3 months later.

155

If this doesn't boggle your mind, maybe this excerpt from "60 MINUTES" will (November 1979) ,in which Mike Wallace interviewed Dr. David Sencer then head of the CDC and the ramrod of the swine flu program.(In our leaders we trust).

Wallace: you began to give the shots in October of '76'?
Dr. Sencer: October 1st.
Wallace: by that time, how many cases of swine flu around the world had been reported?
Dr. Sencer: There had been several reported, but none confirmed. There had been cases in Australia that were reported by the press, by the news media. There were cases in ….
Wallace: None confirmed? Did you ever uncover any other outbreaks of swine flu anywhere in the world?
Dr. Sencer: No
Wallace: Now, nearly everyone was to receive a shot in a public health facility where a doctor might not be present, therefore it was up to the CDC to come up with some kind of official consent form giving the public all the information it needed about the swine flu shot. This form stated that the swine flu vaccine had been tested. What it didn't say was that after those tests were completed, the scientists developed another vaccine and that it was the one given to most of the 46 million who took the shot. That vaccine was called "X-53a". Was X-53a ever field tested?
Dr. Sencer: I-I can't say. I would have to …
Wallace: It wasn't
Dr. Sencer: I don't know.
Wallace: Well, I would think that you're in charge of the program.
Dr. Sencer: I would have to check the records. I haven't looked at this in some time.

Wallace: Did anyone ever come to you and say, "You know something fellows, there's the possibility of neurological damage if you get into a mass immunization program?"

Dr. Sencer: No

Wallace: No one ever did?

Dr. Sencer: No

Wallace: Do you know Michael Hattwick?

Dr. Sencer: Yes, uh-hmm.

Wallace: Dr. Michael Hattwick directed the surveillance team for the swine flu program at the CDC. His job was to find out what possible complications could arise from taking the shot and to report his findings to those in charge. Did you know ahead of time, Dr. Hattwick that there had been case reports of neurological disorders, neurological illness, apparently associated with the injection of influenza vaccine?

Dr. Michael Hattwick: absolutely

Wallace: you did?

Dr. Hattwick: yes

Wallace: how did you know that?

Dr. Hattwick: by review of the literature.

Wallace: so you told your superiors - the men in charge of the swine flu immunization program - about the possibility of neurological disorders?

Dr. Hattwick: Absolutely

Wallace: What would you say if I told you that your superiors say that you never told them about the possibility of neurological complications?

Dr. Hattwick: That's nonsense. I can't believe that they would say that they did not know that there were neurological illnesses associated with influenza vaccination. That simply is not true. We did know that.

Dr. Sencer: I have said that Dr. Hattwick had never told me of his feelings on this subject.

Wallace: Then He's lying?

Dr. Sencer: I guess you would have to make that assumption.

Wallace: Then why does this report from your own agency, dated July 1976, list neurological complications as a possibility.

Dr. Sencer: I think the consensus of the scientific community was that the evidence relating neurological disorders to influenza immunization was such that they did not feel that this association was a real one.

Wallace: You didn't feel it was necessary to tell the American people that information

Dr. Sencer: I think that over the - the years we have tried to inform the American people as - as fully as possible.

Wallace: As part of informing Americans about the swine flue threat, Dr. Sencer's CDC also helped create the advertising to get the public to take the shot. Let me read to you from one of your own agency's memos planning the campaign to urge Americans to take the shot. "The swine flu vaccine has been taken by many important persons," he wrote. "Example: President Ford, Henry Kissinger, Elton John, Muhammad Ali, Mary Tyler Moore, Rudolf Nureyev, Walter Cronkite, Ralph Nader, Edward Kennedy" -etcetera, etcetera, True?

Dr. Sencer: I'm not familiar with that particular piece of paper, but I do know that, at least of that group, President Ford did take the vaccination.

As of 2005 more than 60% of elderly in U.S. receive a yearly Flu shot. This brings us to another troubling association---Influenza Vaccines and Alzheimer's disease.

Prior to the 1976 swine flu vaccine given to 46 million Americans the incidence of Alzheimer's disease in the U.S. population was 0.1 per 100,000 persons From that point the rise in this disease has been precipitous, reaching 10 per 100,000 cases in 2005--a hundredfold increase.

This happens to match very closely with a similar precipitous rise in Autism noted previously. As is the case with Autism the CDC is extremely diligent in avoiding any definitive studies comparing vaccinated with unvaccinated and equivalent groups, which would resolve the issue in both instances appropriately. A single deletion of a useless vitamin study would do the trick.

One of the world's leading immunologists Hugh Fudenburg M.D. (850 papers in peer review journals) had this to say in a speech at the NVIC International vaccine conference, September 1997:
"If an individual has had 5 consecutive flu shots from 1970-1980(the years of the study) his or her chance of developing Alzheimer's disease is 10 times greater than if they had one, two or none.

Despite this highly suggestive evidence, as well as the more recent compelling evidence relating to the total absence of efficacy of flu vaccines previously cited, a noted Mayo clinic Neurologist Brad Boeve M.D. had this to say: (note the usual condescending and snotty tone implying that all criticism is venal and dangerous. Certainly no suggestion that a properly conducted clinical trial might be warranted passed his lips)
"There is absolutely no evidence that flu vaccines contribute in any way to Alzheimer's disease.
If this theory keeps one person from getting the vaccine, and then he or she becomes very ill or dies from the flu, those who write or support such claims have contributed to that person's illness or death."

Thus I stand accused--We have his opinion-- there is no evidence and we don't need any stinking clinical trials!

Finally, a 2005 study published in the Lancet demonstrated that simple hand washing with soap can prevent diarrhea and lower respiratory infection, the two clinical syndromes responsible for the largest number of childhood deaths globally.

There was a more than 50% lower incidence of pneumonia, diarrhea and impetigo in households that received plain soap and hand washing promotion than among controls.

It seems obvious therefore, that a soap and hand washing promotion program is far superior to a ten billion dollar flu vaccine program and is totally without adverse effects.

We have now looked at the cascade effect that was created by Henny Penny. Fortunately, the sky is not falling and influenza deaths, despite claims otherwise by the CDC, are negligible. The "imminent" arrival of the avian flu pandemic has not yet occurred and the millions of stock-piled doses of Tamiflu have now expired and are due to be discarded and replaced.

What we have seen in this chapter should open our eyes a little wider as we move into the broader and darker subject of the world wide vaccine agenda.

CHAPTER XVII
THE VACCINE AGENDA

It should now have become apparent that, at the very least, a systematic collusion involving all the elements of the medical industry exists. This cooperative effort allows a plethora of useless drugs to enter the market-place in a continuous fashion to maintain wind-fall cash profits. A vital part of this process must be the maintenance of a completely closed system with all parties in lock- step. No criticism or alternate technologies are allowed.

The extent to which they have succeeded in this is truly astounding. The ubiquitous pronouncements of medical policy makers in total support of all policies and pharmaceutical agendas are echoed up and down the line. Over and over they preach the line of total efficacy and total safety despite the glaringly obvious data proving otherwise.

We are now entering into this "steel curtain" system at an exponential level that suggests the existence of higher agendas even beyond profit.

Vaccines have become the untouchable holy grail of medicine. No questions allowed. No criticisms broached. The only mantra is safe - safe - safe and more - more - more. The possibility that forty vaccines or fifty or two hundred might be too much for an infant's immune system to tolerate is discarded out of hand.

As we shall see, the vaccine lobby is a huge network of single minded researchers, bureaucrats, politicians, drug company executives, medical institutes and doctors that extend total control into every country and every hospital on earth. There are constant and ongoing meetings at the highest levels involving ministers of health and drug company executives to negotiate contracts involving the proliferation of vaccines world wide.

The CDC through its advisory committees rubber-stamps all vaccines programs put forward by the drug companies. All such advisory committees maintain close financial ties with these companies as they mandate vaccine

162

use and provide a captive base for continuous drug company's profits.

Our task then, is to answer the following questions as definitively as possible:

1. Are vaccines as safe as we are assured?
2. Are vaccines effective as well as cost effective?
3. Do vaccines serve alternate and surreptitious agendas?
4. Are effective antiviral drugs boycotted to protect the vaccine agenda?
5. Who might be the moving parties involved in such a hidden agenda?
6. Can studies ever be allowed that casts doubt on vaccine safety-- leading to huge liabilities?

These questions will be explored and you the reader must assume a position as an advisory committee member to the CDC. When all the facts are in you must make the final judgment. Don't make the mistake of assuming they know much more than you--because they don't.

Much of what we must look at are numbers. Numbers tell the tale and the vaccine cabal feels relatively secure that their "pronouncements" will suffice, and the numbers will never see the light of day. Certainly a review of the data on hundreds of vaccines is well beyond the scope of this book. We will however, take a good look at a representative group of examples, as we did with the influenza vaccine.

To make it clear that the placid acceptance of the vaccine agenda is not universal, it will be useful to quote some dissenting studies and opinions. Antagonism to vaccines is not, as the industry would like to portray, limited to a few (crackpots) who don't happen to be as clever as the experts from the NIH and CDC. They are a large group of credible scientists and researchers who happen not to be on the payroll of the pharmaceutical industry.

163

Bart Classen, a Maryland physician, published data showing that diabetes rates rose significantly in New Zealand following a massive hepatitis B vaccine campaign in young children, and that diabetes rates also went up sharply in Finland after three new childhood vaccines were introduced.

Rebecca Carley, M. D. - "if children receive all recommended vaccines they will receive 2370 times the allowed safe limit for mercury in the first 2 years of life."

Dr. Boyd Haley, professor and chair, Department of Chemistry, University of Kentucky - "a single vaccine given to a 6 pound newborn is the equivalent of giving a 180 pound adult 30 vaccinations on the same day."

Aluminum compounds have been widely used as adjuvants in prophylactic and therapeutic vaccines. Dr. R.K. Gherardi identified a condition known as macrophagic myofascitis causing profound weakness and multiple neurological symptoms. Both human studies and animal studies have shown a strong causal relationship to the aluminum used as a vaccine adjuvant.

The Institute of Medicine in 2004 held a meeting to review research which linked Thimerosal, a mercury - based preservative in vaccines, and neurodevelopmental disorders, such as autism. The panel used data from the centers for disease control (CDC) vaccine data link, which concluded that children who are given 3 Thimerosal containing vaccines are 27 times more likely to develop autism than children who receive Thimerosal-free vaccines.

In October 1988 France became the first country to end hepatitis B vaccination requirements for school children, after reports that many children were developing chronic arthritis and symptoms resembling multiple sclerosis following the administration of the vaccine.

Bonnie Dunbar, PhD. A Texas Cell biologist and vaccine researcher, says, "It takes weeks and sometimes months for autoimmune disorders such as rheumatoid arthritis to develop following vaccination. No basic scientific research or controlled long term studies into the side effects of this vaccine have been conducted on American babies, children, or adults."

For a 20 month period between November 1990 and July 1992 there were 4227 reports of adverse effects from the hepatitis vaccine. The FDA estimates that only 10% of doctors report vaccine injuries and deaths.
Dr. Viera Scheidner, PhD.: "I did not find it difficult to conclude that there is no evidence what-so-ever that vaccines of any kind are effective in preventing the infectious diseases they are supposed to prevent. Furthermore, adverse effects are amply documented and are far more significant to public health than any adverse effect of infectious disease."

A study by New Zealand researchers published in the November 1997 J.of Epidemiology analyzed the health of 1255 children born in 1977:
Of these, 23 didn't get any childhood vaccinations and none of them suffered childhood asthma. Among the 1242 that got polio and DPT shots more than 23% later had episodes of asthma.

Testimony of Bernard Rimland, PhD. Before the House Committee on Government Reform - April 2000:
"Autism is not the only severe chronic illness which has reached epidemic proportions as the number of vaccines has rapidly increased. Children now receive nearly 40 vaccine injections before they enter school - a huge increase. The vaccines contain not only live viruses, but also very significant amounts of highly toxic substances such as mercury, aluminum and formaldehyde. Could this be the reason for the

up surge in autism, ADHD, asthma, arthritis, crohn's disease, lupus and other chronic disorders?" (Not to mention Alzheimer's disease)

Dr. J. Anthony Morris, formally Chief Vaccine Control Officer at the US Federal Drug Administration: "there is a great deal of evidence to prove that immunization of children does more harm than good."

Medical historian Harris Coulter and vaccine researcher Barbara Loe Fisher presented evidence to show that disabilities caused by vaccines are often "disguised" under different names: autism, dyslexia, learning disability, epilepsy, mental retardation, hyperactivity and minimal brain dysfunction. Coulter suggests further linkages to the increase in adolescent crime and suicide, and the decline in SAT scores.

Testimony of vaccine researcher Barbara Loe Fisher PhD. to California Legislature:

"personally, I come here as a parent of a son who had a neurological reaction to his fourth DPT shot at age 2.5 that caused brain dysfunction, including multiple learning disabilities and attention deficit disorder, but who was fortunate not to lose his life or be left with mental retardation, uncontrolled epilepsy, autism, or other severe disabilities like so many of the vaccine injured children I have come to know.

When my son had his vaccine reaction in 1980, children in America were told to get 23 doses of 7 vaccines. Today, children are told to get 37 doses of 11 vaccines. In those 22 years since my son had his vaccine reaction, the numbers of American children with learning disabilities, attention deficit disorder and asthma have doubled; diabetes has tripled: and the incidence of autism has reached epidemic proportions, marking a staggering 2400% increase in the prevalence of autism in our children.

JON RAPPOPORT INTERVIEW OF AN EX VACCINE RESEARCHER

Q: you were once certain that vaccines were the hallmark of good medicine.

A: Yes I was. I helped develop a few vaccines. I won't say which ones.

Q: Why not?

A: I want to preserve my privacy.

Q: So you think you could have problems if you came out into the open?

A: I believe I could lose my pension.

Q: On what grounds?

A: The grounds don't matter. These people have ways of causing you problems, when you were once part of the Club. I know one or two people who were put under surveillance, who were harassed. I was "part of the inner circle." If now I began to name names and make specific accusations against researcher, I could be in a world of trouble.

Q: What is at the bottom of these efforts at harassment?

A: Vaccines are the last defense of modern medicine. Vaccines are the ultimate justification for the overall "brilliance" of modern medicine.

Q: Do you believe that people should be allowed to choose whether they should get vaccines?

A: On a political level, yes. On a scientific level, people need information, so that they can choose well. Its one thing to say choice is good. But if the atmosphere is full of lies, how can you choose? Also, if the FDA were run by honorable people, these vaccines would not be granted licenses. They would be investigated to within an inch of their lives.

Q: There are medical historians who state that the overall decline of illnesses was not due to vaccines.

A: I know. For a long time, I ignored their work.

Q: Why?

A: Because I was afraid of what I would find out. I was in the business of developing vaccines. My livelihood depended on continuing that work.

167

Q: And then?

A: I did my own investigation.

Q: What conclusions did you come to?

A: The decline of disease is due to improved living conditions.

Q: What conditions?

A: Cleaner water. Advanced sewage systems. Nutrition, fresher food. A decrease in poverty. Germs may be everywhere, but when you are healthy, you don't contract the diseases as easily.

Q: What did you feel when you completed your own investigation?

A: Despair. I realized I was working a sector based on a collection of lies.

Q: are some vaccines more dangerous than others?

A. Yes. The DPT shot, for example. The MMR. But some lots of vaccine are more dangerous than others. lots of the same vaccine. As far as I'm concerned, all vaccines are dangerous.

Q: Why?

A: Several reasons. They involve the human immune system in a process that tends to compromise immunity. They can actually cause the disease they are supposed to prevent. They can cause other diseases than the ones they are supposed to prevent.

Q: Why are we quoted statistics which seem to prove that vaccines have been tremendously successful at wiping out diseases?

A: Why? To give the illusion that these vaccines are useful. If a vaccine suppresses visible symptoms of a disease like measles, everyone assumes that the vaccine is a success. But, under the surface, the vaccine can harm the immune system itself. And if its causes other diseases --say, meningitis-- that fact is masked, because no one believes that the vaccine can do that. The connection is overlooked.

Q: It is said that the smallpox vaccine wiped out smallpox in England.

A: Yes. But when you study the available statistics, you get another picture.

Q: Which is?

A: There were cities in England where people who were not vaccinated did not get smallpox. There were places where people who were vaccinated experienced smallpox epidemics. And smallpox was already on the decline before the vaccine was introduced.

Q: So you're saying that we have been treated to a false history.

A: Yes. That's exactly what I'm saying. This is a history that has been cooked up to convince people that vaccines are invariably safe and effective.

Q: Now, you worked in labs. Where purity was an issue.

A: The public believes that these labs, these manufacturing facilities are the cleanest places in the world. That is not true. Contamination occurs all the time. You get all sorts of debris introduced into vaccines.

Q: For example, the SV40 monkey virus slips into the polio vaccine.

A: Well yes, that happened. But that's not what I mean. The SV40 got into the polio vaccine because the vaccine was made by using monkey kidneys. But I'm talking about something else. The actual lab conditions. The mistakes. The careless errors. SV40, which was later found in cancer tumors--that was what I would call a structural problem. It was an accepted part of the manufacturing process. If you use monkey kidney, you open the door to germs which you don't know are in the kidneys.

Q: Okay, but let's ignore that distinction between different types of contaminants for a moment. What contaminants did you find in your many years of work with vaccines?

A: All right. I'll give you some of what I came across, and I'll also give you what colleagues of mine found. Here's a partial list. In the Rimavex measles vaccine, we found various chicken viruses. In polio vaccine, we found acanthameoba, which is a so-called "brain-eating" amoeba.

Simian cytomegalovirus in polio vaccine. Simian foamy virus in the rotavirus vaccine. Bird-cancer viruses in the MMR vaccine. Various micro-organisms in the anthrax vaccine. I've found potentially dangerous enzyme inhibitors in several vaccines. Duck, dog, and rabbit viruses in the rubella vaccine. Avian leucosis virus in the flu vaccine. Pestivirus in the MMR vaccine.

Q: Alarm bells are ringing all over the place.

A: How do you think I felt? Remember, this material is going into the blood stream without passing through some of the ordinary immune defenses.

Q: How were you findings received?

A: Basically, it was, don't worry, this can't be helped. In making vaccines, you use various animals" tissue, and that's where this kind of contamination enters in. Of course, I'm not even mentioning the standard chemicals like formaldehyde, mercury, and aluminum which are purposely put into vaccines.

Q: This information is pretty staggering.

A: Yes. And I'm just mentioning some of the biological contaminants. Who knows how many others there are? Others we don't find because we don't think to look for them. If tissues from, say, a bird is used to make a vaccine, how many possible germs can be in that tissue? We have no idea. We have no idea what they might be, or what effects they could have on humans.

Q: And beyond the purity issue?

A: You are dealing with the basic faulty premise about vaccines. That they intricately stimulate the immune system to create the conditions for immunity from disease. That is the bad premise. It doesn't work that way. A vaccine is supposed to "create" antibodies which, indirectly, offer protection against disease, however, the immune system is much larger and more involved than antibodies and their related "killer cells."

Q: In your years working in the vaccine establishment, how many doctors did you encounter who admitted that vaccines were a problem?

A: None. There were a few who privately questioned what they were doing. But they would never go public, even within their companies.

Q: What was the turning point for you?

A: I had a friend whose baby died after a DPT shot.

Q: Did you investigate?

A: Yes, informally. I found this baby was completely healthy before the vaccination. There was no reason for his death, except the vaccine. That started my doubts. Of course, I wanted to believe that the baby had gotten a bad shot from a bad lot. But as I looked into this further, I found that was not the case in this instance. I was being drawn into a spiral of doubt that increased over time. I continued to investigate. I found that, contrary to what I thought, vaccines are not tested in a scientific way.

Q: What do you mean?

A: For example, no long-term studies are done on any vaccines. Long-term follow-up is not done in any careful way. Why? Because, again, the assumption is made that vaccines do not cause problems. So why should anyone check? On top of that, a vaccine reaction is defined so that all bad reactions are said to occur very soon after the shot is given. But that does not make sense.

Q: Why doesn't it made sense?

A: Because the vaccine obviously acts in the body for a long period of time after it is given. A reaction can be gradual. Deterioration can be gradual. Neurological problems can develop over time. They do in various conditions, even according to a Conventional analysis. So why couldn't that be the case with vaccines? If chemical poisoning can occur gradually, why couldn't that be the case with a vaccine which contains mercury?

Q: And that is what you found?

A: Yes. You are dealing with correlations, most of the time. Correlations are not perfect. But if you get 500 parents whose children have suffered neurological damage during a one-year period after having a vaccine, this should be sufficient to spark off an intense investigation.

Q: Has it been enough?

A: No. Never. This tells you something right away.

Q: Which is?

A: The people doing the investigation are not really interested in looking at the facts. They assure that the vaccines are safe. So, when they do investigate, they invariably come up with exonerations of the vaccines. They say, "This vaccine is safe." But what do they base those judgments on? They base them on definitions and ideas which automatically rule out a condemnation of the vaccine.

Q: What about the combined destructive power of a number of vaccines given to babies these days?

A: It is a travesty and a crime. There are no real studies of any depth which have been done on that. Again, the assumption is made that vaccines are safe, and therefore any number of vaccines given together are safe as well. But the truth is vaccines are not safe. Therefore the potential damage increases when you give many of them in a short time period.

Q: Then we have the fall flu season.

A: Yes. As if only in the autumn do these germs float into the US from Asia. The public swallows that premise. If it happens in April, it is a bad cold. If it happens in October it is the flu.

Q: Do you regret having worked all those years in the vaccine field?

A: Yes. But after this interview, I'll regret it a little less. And I work in other ways. I give out information to certain people, when I think they will use it well.

Q: What is one thing you want the public or understand?

A: That the burden or proof in establishing the safety and efficacy of vaccines is on the people who manufacture and license them for public use. Just that. The burden of proof is not on you or me. And for proof you need well-designed long-term studies. You need extensive follow-up. You need to interview mothers and pay attention to what mothers say about their babies and what happens to them after vaccination. You need all these things. The things that are not there.

EXCERPTS FROM AN ARTICLE BY ROBERT F. KENNEDY JR.:
THE THIMEROSAL SCANDAL

Mounting evidence suggests that Thimerosal, a preservative in many children's vaccines that breaks down to release the neurotoxin ethyl mercury, may be responsible for the exponential growth of autism and other childhood neurological disorders now epidemic in the United States.

Some scientists believe that Thimerosal in children's inoculations may even be the cause of the hundred-point loss in Scholastic Aptitude Scores among children born in the "Thimerosal generation."

The ethyl mercury released from Thimerosal is a known neural poison and autism rates began rising dramatically in children who were administrated the new vaccine regimen. A decade ago, the American Academy of Pediatrics estimated the autism rate among American children to be 1 in 2500. Today, both the AAP and the CDC place the autism rate at an astonishing 1 in 166, or 1 in 80 boys! Additionally, 1 in every 6 children is now diagnosed with a related neurological disorder.

In May of 1999, Patti White, RN, submitted her testimony to the Government Reform Committee, giving the school nurses perspective on the growing epidemic.
"the elementary grades are overwhelmed with children who have symptoms of neurological and /or immune system damage; epilepsy, seizure disorders, palsies, autism, mental retardation, learning disabilities, diabetes, asthma,

173

vision/hearing loss, and a multiplicity of new conduct/behavior disorders. We (school nurses) have come to believe that vaccines are an assault on a new-born's developing neural and immune system. Vaccines are supposed to be making us healthier; however, in 25 years of nursing I have never seen so many damaged, sick kids. **Something very, very wrong is happening to our children." There are now 1.5 million autistics in the United States with 40 thousand new cases each year.**

During the 1990's, there were a significant number of reports filed into VAERS (the vaccine adverse reporting system) from doctors and parents of children who's autism seemed directly linked to vaccines. In response, the CDC asked its employee Thomas Verstraeten to perform the first live study of over one hundred thousand American children whose vaccine and medical records were stored in the CDC's vaccine safety data link (VSD).

Verstraeten provoked alarm within the vaccine industry community when his data showed clear causative link between Thimerosal and neurological damage, including autism. "The harm", Verstraeten observed, "is done in the first month of life by Thimerosal in vaccines."

He wrote in a December 1999 email to Robert Davis, a leading pharmaceutical industry consultant, that despite "running, rethinking, rerunning, and rethinking" the damaging effect of Thimerosal persisted. He titled his 1999 email, "it just won't go away."

When Thomas Saari, a spoke-person for the American Academy of Pediatrics reviewed Verstraeten's data, he panicked. "What if the lawyers get a hold of this?" He wrote in an email to his colleagues, "There's not a scientist in the world that can refute these findings."

As word of Verstraeten's findings spread, panicked public health agencies that had green-lighted Thimerosal began warning each other of the study's implications. In a

174

June 1999 e-mail memo to the CDC's Jose Cordero and Robert Bernier, Peter Patriarca, the director of FDA's Division of Viral Products and an American Association of Pediatrics Infectious Diseases Committee member (both AAP and FDA had strongly supported the vaccine regimen), worried that "the greatest point of vulnerability on this issue is that the systematic review of Thimerosal in vaccines by the FDA could have been done years ago. The calculations done by FDA are not complex.)By then, the FDA had calculated that a birth dose of the hepatitis B vaccine would result in mercury exposure nearly 38 times the EPA safety guideline. Referring to huge cumulative doses of Thimerosal that children were now receiving in the multiple vaccinations. Patriarca observed, "we must keep in mind the dose of ethyl mercury was not generated by rocket science (It) involves ninth grade algebra. What took the FDA so long to do the calculations? Why didn't CDC and the advisory bodies do these calculations when they rapidly expanded the childhood immunization schedule?" He added, "I'm not sure if there will be an easy way out of the potential perception that the FDA, CDC and immunization policy bodies may have been asleep at the wheel re. Thimerosal until now.

Then Patriarca pointed out the seminal problem that helped provoke this public health crisis in the first place, and that would steer government officials into a shameful conspiracy to cover up the greatest public health scandal in American history; the ubiquitous conflicts of interest, financial and otherwise--that infect relationships between the pharmaceutical industry and the public health authorities. "It will also raise questions," he cautioned, "about various advisory bodies regarding aggressive recommendations for the use of Thimerosal in child vaccines."

Many members on the advisory bodies who review vaccine science have financial ties to industry. The agencies tainted by these conflicts include the Centers for Disease

175

Control and prevention ("CDC"), the agency charged with investigating medical issues; the Food and Drug Administration ("FDA"), the agency charged with regulating vaccines; the Institute of Medicine ("IOM"), which examines policy issues for the National Academies; and the American Academy of Pediatrics (AAP).

Of these, CDC is particularly compromised. CDC has the extraordinary power to guarantee a market and profit to vaccine makers. But the people make these decisions often have a financial stake in their outcomes. According to a February 2004 report by UPI investigative journalist Mark Benjamin, members of CDC's vaccine advisory committees often share vaccine patents, own stock in vaccine companies, receive payment for research or to monitor vaccine trials, and funding for academic departments.

Furthermore, CDC itself each year receives money from vaccine makers from licensing agreements and for work on collaborative projects and CDC scientists regularly leave the agency to work for vaccine manufacturers.

For example, officials on the committee that mandated the Thimerosal-laden hepatitis B vaccination for infants in 1991 were closely tied to industry. The advisory committee chair, Sam Katz, helped develop a measles vaccine manufactured by Merck, which also manufactures the hepatitis B vaccine. When he chaired the committee, he was also a paid consultant for Merck, Wyeth and most of the other vaccine makers. Another member of that committee was Dr. Neal Halsey, Director of the Division of Disease Control at John Hopkins University and former CDC employee. Halsey has worked as a consultant and researcher for most of the vaccine companies. His Institute for Vaccine Safety at Johns Hopkins is funded by vaccine manufacturers including Merck and Wyeth.

An August 2001 report by the House Government Reform Committee found that "four out of eight CDC advisory committee members who voted to approve guidelines for the rotavirus vaccine in June 1998 had financial ties to the pharmaceutical companies that were developing different versions of the vaccine. One of them was Dr. Paul Offit, who shared a patent for one of the rotavirus vaccines and acknowledged he would make money if the vaccines were approved.

Despite his professed best effort to manipulate the data to reduce the effect, Verstraeten's confidential report of February 2000 concluded that there was a 10 fold increased risk of autism and related neurodevelopmental problems, resulting from the mercury in the vaccine.

He shared his findings that month at a secret meeting with 60 pharmaceutical industry representatives and public health officials at the Simpsonwood Retreat center in Norcross, Georgia. The meeting was held with no public notice and apparently convened at Simpsonwood to avoid the reach of the Freedom of Information laws which pubic health officials interpreted to cover only meetings at government offices.

Attendees included numerous high ranking CDC and FDA representatives, vaccine officials from WHO (World Health Organization), and representatives of vaccine makers GlaxoSmithKline, Merck, and Aventis, all of whom are named defendants in lawsuits by the parents of autistic children.

Transcripts of those discussions were first obtained by a Congressional committee investigating Thimerosal and more recently by Safe Minds, a group of anti-Thimerosal advocates. Those transcripts paint an unsavory picture of frantic scrambling by vaccine makers and CDC reps that had seen Verstraeten's unpublished study. We see leaders at the highest level of America's medical community charged with protecting public health, hatching a plan with pharmaceuticals to hide the dangers of Thimerosal from the public, and to protect the pharmaceutical manufacturers and the regulatory agency bureaucrats who had approved its use, from liability.

Dr. Verstraeten, who shortly after that meeting announced that he had accepted a job working for Thimerosal vaccine maker GlaxoSmithKline, introduced his research as "the study that nobody thought we should do," and summarized his findings; "we have found statistically significant relationships between" Thimerosal exposure and neurological disorders. He noted that "the bottom line ...our signal [linking Thimerosal to neurological disorders] will simply not go away. He warned that even this thoroughly damming data actually understates the true problem, because many of the children considered in the study were "just not old enough to be diagnosed," (autism is typically not diagnosed until age three or four) and predicted that the problem in this cohort would certainly get worse.

Dr. Verstraeten recounted that the clear relationship between Thimerosal and autism and other neurological disorders reflected in the VSD data had prompted him to review the large body of research studies linking Thimerosal to brain damage. "When I saw this, and I went back through the literature, I was actually stunned by what I saw".

Dr. John Clements, an advisor to the Vaccines and Biologics division of the World Health Organization, and an aggressive advocate of Thimerosal-laced vaccines in Third World nations, also tipped his hat to the wide body of existing studies linking Thimerosal and neurological disorders while remonstrating those members of the group who had allowed Verstraeten's research to proceed, flatly declaring "this study should not have been done at all, because the outcome of it could have, to some extent, been predicted." No matter what steps the committee takes now to mitigate Verstraeten's inescapable conclusions, he warned that "through freedom of information laws, Verstraeten's work will be taken by others and will be used in other ways beyond the control of this group." And he urged that "now the research results have to be handled."

The meeting closed with a discussion about how to keep the information from the public. "We have been privileged so far, that given the sensitivity of information, we have been able to manage to keep it out of, let's say, less responsible hands," said Bob Chen, head of CDC's Vaccine Safety and Development unit." Consider this embargoed information," Dr Roger Bernier, the associate director for Science at the CDC's National Immunization Program (NIP) announced at the meeting's close. "We have asked you to keep this information confidential...while we..consider these data in a certain protected environment."

Verstraeten's initial study was never published and the CDC scrambled to block public access to his original data and the Vaccine Safety Datalink (VSD) files in general. In 2002, CDC turned its VSD data files over to an outside agency, the American Association of Health Plans, with a $190 million contract that purports to shield the data from Sunshine Laws like the Freedom of information Act (FOIA) or even subpoena, by characterizing the data as proprietary to the HMO's that helped generate it. CDC has told independent researchers that Verstraeten's original data has been lost, and that there is no way to replicate his original study. This despite the fact that iron-clad ethical standards dictate that agencies like CDC retain scientific research data so that it can be replicated.

The CDC then commissioned the Institute of Medicine (IOM) to develop its own assessment of the link between Thimerosal and neurological disorders. CDC and NIH funded the review with over $2 million and worked in collaboration with IOM to develop its conclusions. Since CDC, as the primary advocate for Thimerosal-containing vaccines and the expanded vaccine schedule, was neck-deep in this tragedy, its involvement in the study presented a clear conflict of interest.

CDC's directives to the IOM from the start were transparent; the new studies should not find a link between

179

Thimerosal and neurological disorders and, regardless of the facts, should reassure the public about vaccine safety.

Dr. Marie McCormick, chair of the Immunization Review Committee, was even more frank, noting that the CDC, which had funded the $2 million study, "wants us to declare, well, these things are pretty safe..." Before her committee reviewed a single study or a shred of data she expressed her confidence that, "we are not ever going to come down that autism is a true side effect of vaccine exposure. Dr. McCormick told me emphatically that she receives no money from the pharmaceutical companies but records show that the Harvard School of Public Health, where she works as a chairperson, receives millions from pharmaceutical companies.

Dr. Kathleen Stratton, a member of IOM staff and study director of the Immunization Safety Review Committee, reiterated McCormick's message, "we said this before you got here, and I think we said this yesterday, the point of no return, the line we will not cross in public policy is to pull the vaccine, change the schedule... We wouldn't say compensate, we wouldn't say pull the vaccine, we wouldn't say stop the program."

Despite not having heard any of the evidence, she predicted that the probable conclusion was going to be that the "evidence was inadequate to accept or reject a causal relation between vaccines and neurological disorders." She said that this result was "what Walt said he wanted." Dr. Stratton told me she was referring to Walter A. Orenstein, M. D., the former Director of the National Immunization Program at the Centers for Disease Control and Prevention (CDC) in Atlanta, Georgia. "Even recommending research is recommendation for policy, "she added, signaling IOM's apparent intent to derail further research on the links between Thimerosal and neurological disorders. When I recently asked Stratton, and then pressed her repeatedly, whether she would give Thimerosal to her own children, she refused to answer the question.

It was an open secret among high-ranking public health officials that the CDC studies were not intended to explore, study or assess the link between Thimerosal and neurological disorders, but to "rule out" any links, and to give cover to official statements that Thimerosal was safe. In May 2001, Dr. Gordon Douglas, M.D., Director of Strategic Planning for the Vaccine Research Center at the National Institutes of Health (NIH) assured a Princeton University gathering that, "Four current studies are taking place at the CDC in collaboration with NIH to rule out the proposed link between autism and Thimerosal." In addition to his federal duties as a leading public health official, Dr. Douglas also works for the Thimerosal vaccine producer Aventis and formerly served as president of Merck's vaccination program. In that capacity in 1991, he had received Dr. Hilleman's urgent warning about Thimerosal and chose to ignore it. With extraordinary candor he told his listeners, "In order to undo the harmful effects of research claiming to link vaccines to an elevated risk of autism, we need to conduct and publicize additional studies.. To assure parents of vaccine safety.

In May 2004, IOM issued its pre-ordained conclusion that there was no proven link between autism and Thimerosal in vaccines and strongly recommended that no further studies should address the issue.

The IOM relied on five badly flawed epidemiological studies. Four of them were from European countries whose populations were exposed to a fraction of the Thimerosal given to American kids, and not initially exposed on the day of birth, but five weeks later.

At the Simpsonwood meeting Dr. Robert Brent had urged investigators "to get other populations to study, arguing that "I do not think that reanalysis of the American data is going to be as helpful as we would hope."

"What we care most about," says a note from one participant "is a consistent body of epidemiological evidence that consistently shows no association." Notes from at least one other committee member indicate that CDC was already planning to use epidemiology from Europe to disprove causation.

All of the key studies relied upon by IOM not only have disastrously flawed methodologies, but most of their authors are burdened with serious conflicts of interest and bias that cast doubt on the integrity of their reports. Most of the conflicts arise from financial ties with the very vaccine makers who are defendants in Thimerosal lawsuits.

Republican Congressman Dave Weldon, M. D., whose Human Rights and Wellness Sub-Committee had been investigating the links between Thimerosal and autism for three years in an exhaustive process that included testimony from numerous scientific experts, immediately attacked the IOM report for its conclusions and the IOM and CDC for their conflicts of interest and bias. Later that month, the Congressional Record published "The Mercury in Medicine Report" -on May21, 2003 by Weldon's committee.

The committee report made specific finding that: "The CDC in general and the National Immunization Program in particular conflicted in their duties to monitor the safety of vaccines, while also charged with the responsibility of purchasing vaccines for resale as well as promoting increased immunization rates."

The report faulted CDC which, it said, was plagued by "biases against theories regarding vaccine-induced autism," had therefore selected researchers "who also worked for vaccine manufactures to conduct population-based epidemiological studies." The report condemned the IOM studies as "of poor design, under-powered, and fatally flawed." The report went on to say:**"Thimerosal used as a preservative in vaccines is likely related to the autism epidemic.** This epidemic in all probability may have been prevented or curtailed had the FDA not been asleep at the switch regarding the lack of safety data regarding injected Thimerosal and the sharp rise of infant exposure to this known neurotoxin. Our public health agencies' fail to act is indicative of institutional malfeasance for self protection and **misplaced protectionism of the pharmaceutical industry.**"

Congressman Weldon told me that there is an extremely close relationship between the CDC and vaccine manufacturers and CDC's treasured "partnerships" with the vaccine industry invariably take precedence over vaccine safety. Weldon explained that CDC is not interested in an honest search for truth on the issue because "an association between vaccines and autism would force CDC officials to admit that their policies irreparably damaged thousands of children. Who would want to make that conclusion about themselves?"

Dr. Boyd Haley adds that if CDC was really interested in uncovering the truth, it would commission epidemiological studies of American cohorts who escaped vaccination, most obviously the children of Jehovah's Witnesses, Christian Scientists or the Amish. But CDC has instead worked furiously to quash such studies by cutting off federal funding and denying independent scientists access to the VSD database. Using that database, scientists could make comparative studies of children receiving zero mercury from vaccines and children that were fully vaccinated. CDC says it made the VSD unavailable to outside researchers due to "potential issues of patient confidentiality." But Haley says that patient confidentiality is routinely safeguarded through a number of well-established techniques in such studies.

When I raised the possibility of encouraging such studies to Kathleen Stratton, the chief IIOM staffer on the Thimerosal panel, she told me. "That's a great idea; no one has ever suggested it before." The statement is incredible; Stratton was the chief scientific organizer of the IOM's vaccine project; the idea of finding an uncontaminated U.S. cohort to study as a "control" group is science 101. In fact, Dr. Boyd Haley has repeatedly urged IOM and CDC to conduct such a study, including at two public and tape-recorded meetings - one of these attended by Kathleen Stratton.

In April 2005, UPI reporter Dan Olmsted undertook the task himself. He scoured the Amish of Lancaster, Pennsylvania, who refused to immunize their infants. Given the national rate of autism, Olmsted calculated that there should be 130 autistics among the Amish. He found only four. One had been exposed to high levels of mercury from a power plant. The other three - including one child adopted from outside the Amish community - had received their vaccines.

We may now be tainting U.S. foreign relations by exporting this scandal to the Third World. In 1999, the federal government began purchasing tens of millions of dollars of Thimerosal-containing vaccines for export to developing countries. At that time autism was virtually unknown in the developing world. Our export of Thimerosal-containing vaccines has been followed by exploding autism rates in India, Argentina and Nicaragua, and other lands where the disease had not previously been reported. At the same time, GlaxoSmithKline and Merck began aggressively marketing Thimerosal-containing vaccines to China's communist government. As David Kirby reports in his new book Evidence of Harm, Mercury in Vaccines and the Autism Epidemic: A Medical Controversy, a few years after the vaccine manufacturers launched their campaign, the number of cases of children suffering from autism "unexpectedly skyrocketed." This past August, Xin Hua, China's news agency, reported that autism rates in China have risen from almost zero previously to 1.8 million cases reported last year. Scientists estimate an astonishing annual growth rate of 20% for the disease in China.

All of this information should raise the question of why the concern of the WHO (World Health Organization) to implement massive world wide vaccine program appears to take precedence over the health of our children. With or without Thimerosal, the vaccine agenda moves inexorably forward without any clear idea of the long term consequences. After all there are thousands of pathogenic organisms that could be targeted by vaccines and are we to accept the consequences of thousands of vaccines in the future? Who might be behind this and might there be a hidden agenda? For that answer we have to go back a few years.

In 1974, Henry Kissinger presented to the National Security Council, memorandum 200 on world population growth and the implications for national security of the United States. This memorandum postulated the measures to be implemented through the coordination of the following institutions:

The World Bank, WHO, UN, UNICEF, and private groups and foundations including the Rockefeller Foundation. Over the ensuing years this identical conglomerate morphed into an entirely different agenda that is now dispersing vaccines to the world.

Spearheaded by the Rockefeller Foundation and now funded by the Bill Gates foundation, this new initiative is known as GAVI or the Global Alliance for Vaccine Immunization.

In this regard, Robert McNamara, the former President of the World Bank, the former United States Secretary of Defense and a member of the expanded program on immunization, made some interesting remarks. "One must take draconian measures of demographic reduction against the will of the population. Reducing the birth rate has proved to be impossible or insufficient. One must therefore increase the mortality rate. How? By natural means. Famine and sickness".

Even further insight into the possibility of hidden agendas can be gleaned from reading between the words and deeds of the Bill and Melinda Gates Foundation.

The story of the Bill and Melinda Gates Foundation may well be the seminal tale of a hidden agenda dressed in sheep's clothing. If we examine the website of the Gates Foundation we find unrestrained homage to the highest motives and priorities. "We support efforts to stop HIV transmission including the developing of a safe, effective and affordable HIV vaccine. In addition, we support the development of microbicides-gels or creams that allow women to protect themselves from HIV infection." The website goes on to explain how prevention efforts could save half of the 60 million new infections expected by the year 2015. The website lists as priority diseases, HIV/AID's, malaria, tuberculosis, diarrhea, respiratory infection and vaccine preventable diseases.

It was recently announced that an anti- HIV gel failed in a key trial funded by the Gates Foundation in a group of 6000 South African women. New infections were equal in the treated and placebo group. The gel used in this study did prove to be safe, however, and researchers referred to that as a "water- shed event". Such a response to total failure after two decades of effort seems inappropriate [in my opinion]. It should be mentioned that the substance tested in this ground breaking trial was seaweed and one might well have expected such a result.

You might at this point be wondering what relevance this has to the topic of this chapter. I will make this very clear shortly. I first wish to point out three salient facts that must be kept in mind.

First is the 20 year failure to develop a prophylactic vaginal gel for HIV. Second ,the provision of more than one billion dollars by Gates to inject every newborn African baby with hepatitis B vaccine on the first day of their lives. Thirdly, that the bulk of the Gates foundations priorities are to be addressed by the use of vaccines.

In regard to the first point, after 20 years of effort one wonders why the culmination is a failed study testing seaweed. As to the second point, no physician that I have queried has been able to explain to me why it is appropriate to spend billions of dollars on newborn hepatitis B vaccinations when hepatitis B is contracted through the use of contaminated needles and by major sexual promiscuity. By the time these babies reach the appropriate age for such activity the protection would surely have long dissipated.

The ostensible rationale put forward by the hepatitis B vaccine proponents is that chronic hepatitis B infection can lead to cirrhosis and ultimately liver cancer in a small percentage of cases. Therefore deaths from liver cancer are preventable by hepatitis B vaccine. Even if this was true, liver cancer is a disease of the elderly, a state unlikely to be reached by any of today's African babies. The billions wasted in this extraordinary effort could save many thousands of babies that will never live long enough to develop liver cancer.

It should be noted that this same hepatitis B vaccine is being used on all newborns in the United States as well. In the year 2007 there were 16 thousand cases of hepato-cellular carcinoma (liver cancer) in the United States. The vast majority were between 60 and 80 years of age. 95% of these cases were due to alcoholism. Somewhere in the remaining 5% were the cases due to hepatitis B along with all the other causes of liver cancer. The reality is that no more than a few hundred deaths can be attributed to chronic hepatitis B infections, far fewer than the deaths and adverse events caused by the vaccine itself.

In a subsequent chapter we will see how hepatitis B vaccine may have been used for an alternate agenda. Meanwhile, in November 2007 in conjunction with KEMRI, the eighth largest Research Institute in the world and the largest such institute in Africa ,I, as Chief Director of Research, presented a carefully crafted application in strict compliance with the Directives of the Gates Foundation for the funding of multiple third stage trials of ALPHAMIR. These trials were to encompass the primary stated priorities of the Gates Foundation, for an effective treatment and prophylactic gel for HIV/AID's as well as for treatment of malaria, tuberculosis, respiratory and diarrheal illnesses-the very priorities enumerated in their website. This request was for 24 million dollars to be used for the entire project over a period over 2 years.

Keep in mind that Alphamir had already been proven and approved for the treatment of HIV and rheumatoid arthritis by the Ministry of Health of Kenya. Also, it should be noted that the Gates Foundation had just remitted an additional 750 million dollars to GAVI for hepatitis B vaccines in Africa.

The following was the response to our request received in January 2008;

To; Stephen Herman, M. D. Chief Research Director, Kenya Medical Research Institute.

Dear Dr. Herman, Thank you for writing to the Bill and Melinda Gates Foundation. Foundation staff was pleased to have an opportunity to review your letter (submission) and to learn about your activities.

We receive a large number of interesting (good choice of words) proposals and unfortunately are unable to fund all of them. We regret that we are unable to provide support for your activities because of competing priorities for resources (read vaccines).

We appreciate your commitment to this work and wish you great success with your endeavor.
Sincerely,
Rachel Jackson
Program Coordinator

Well, quelle surprise! Competing priorities indeed. What puts HIV, HIV microbicide, malaria and tuberculosis way down on the list of priorities? Simply this - vaccines! It seemed that an alternate technology for the treatment of viral disease is not going to be allowed to interfere with the vaccine agenda.

NEW SCIENTIST ARTICLE APRIL 2006
STOCKPILE HUMAN BIRD FLU VACCINE NOW SAY EXPERTS
The US plans to spend 1.2 billion on a pre-pandemic vaccine and the UK announced it would buy 2 million doses.

In as much as the vaccine against seasonal flu has proven useless, the plan now is to sell billions of dollars worth of bird flu vaccine which surely would be equally as worthless against the so far non-existent bird flu pandemic. If the avian flu virus were to mutate, so as to be infectious between individual humans, surely this degree of mutation would render any vaccine useless.

This reality has certainly not escaped the proponents of such a pre- pandemic vaccine. Also, they know that a truly effective anti- viral could interfere with their vaccine agenda; they also know that a totally ineffective anti-viral, such as Tamiflu, is perfectly acceptable and should be stockpiled. An ineffective drug doesn't interfere with anything.

Certainly the Gates Foundation can't claim ignorance or stupidity. What's really going on? Perhaps an article in the LA Times might be enlightening;

DARK CLOUD OVER GATES FOUNDATION

"Like most philanthropies, the Gates Foundation gives away at least 5% of its worth every year, to avoid paying most taxes. In 2005, it granted nearly 1.4 billion dollars. It awards grants

189

mainly in support of global health initiatives. It invests the other 95% of its worth. This endowment is managed by Bill Gates Investments, which handles Gates' personal fortune.

The Times found that the Gates Foundations endowment had major holdings in:

- Companies ranked among the worst US and Canadian polluters, including Conoco Phillips, Dow Chemical Corp and Tyco International Ltd.

- Many of the worlds worst polluters, including companies that own an oil refinery and one that owns a paper mill, which a study shows, sicken children while the foundation tries to save their parents from AIDS.

- Pharmaceutical companies that price drugs beyond the reach of AID's patients the foundation is trying to treat. (And that manufacture vaccines)

Using the most recent data available, a Times tally showed that hundreds of Gates foundation investments- totaling at least 8.7 billion dollars - have been in companies that countered the foundations charitable goals or socially concerned philosophy.

This is "the dirty secret" of many large philanthropies, said Paul Hawken, an expert on socially beneficial investing who directs the Natural Capital Institute, an investment research group. "Foundations donate to groups trying to heal the future,"Hawken said in an interview, "but with their investments, they steal from their future".

At a clinic in Isipingo, a suburb of the South African port city of Durban, where the HIV infection rate is as high 40%, Pembeka Dube age 20 was getting a checkup. Dube had volunteered for tests of a vaginal gel that researchers hoped would be shown to protect against HIV. The test was part of a study conducted by the New York based Population Council and funded by a 20 million dollar grant from the Bill and Melinda Gates Foundation.

Dube's boyfriend won't use condoms. She hoped the tests would show she could use the microbicidal gel, called

Carraguard, and stop worrying about AIDS. (Following the failure of this seaweed derivative the Gates Foundation still found KEMRI's technology, Alphamir, of too low a priority to consider?).

Research into prophylactics such as Carraguard can fight AIDS by empowering women, Bill Gates told the International AIDS Conference in Toronto in August. "Whether the woman is a faithful married mother of small children, or a sex worker trying to scrape out a living in a slum..." he said, "a woman should never need her partner's permission to save her own life."

Two days before Gates spoke; Kyrone Smith was born, a few kilometers from the Isipingo Clinic. At the same time the Gates Foundation was trying to help Dube with its seaweed microbicide, it owned a stake in companies that appeared to be hurting Kyrone.

At 6 weeks, his lungs began to fail. Kyrone struggled to cry, but he was so weak that no sound came out - just husky, labored breath.

His mother, Renee Smith, 26, rushed him to a hospital, where he was given oxygen. She feared it would be the first of many hospital visits. Smith knew from experience.

"My son Teiago was in and out of the hospital since the age of three," she said. "He couldn't breathe nicely... There are so many children in this area who have the same problems."

Two of the areas worst industrial polluters- the Mondi Paper Mill and a giant SAPREF Oil Refinery-squat among the homes near Isipingo like sleepy grey dragons, exhaling chemical vapors day and night. The SAPREF Plant, which has had 2 dozen significant spills, flares, pipeline ruptures and explosions since 1998 and the Mondi Plant together pump thousands of tons putrid-smelling chemicals into the air annually, according to their own monitoring.

In 2002, a study found that more than half of the children at a school in nearby Merebank suffered asthma--one of the highest rates in scientific literature. A second study, published last year, found serious respiratory problems throughout the region; more than half of children age 2 to 5 had asthma, largely attributed to sulfur dioxide and other industrial pollutants. Much of it was produced by companies in which the Gates Foundation was invested.

Asthma was not the only danger. Isipingo is in what environmental activists called "cancer valley." Emissions of benzene, dioxins and other carcinogens were "among the highest levels found in any comparable location in the world," said Stewart Batterman at the University of Michigan, a co-author of both studies.

The Gates Foundation is a major shareholder in the company that owns both of the polluting plants. As of September the foundation held 295 million dollars worth of stock in BP, a co-owner of SAPREF. As of 2005, it held 35 million dollars worth of stock in Royal Dutch Shell, SAPREF's other owner. The Foundation also holds a 39 million dollar investment in Anglo- American, which owns the Mondi Paper Mill.

The Foundation has gotten much more in financial gain from its investments in the polluters than it has given to the Durbin microbicide study to fight AIDS.

Just as the Gates Foundations investments in Mondi, BP and Royal Dutch Shell have been very profitable, so to have its holdings in the top 100 polluters in the United States, as rated by the University of Massachusetts, and the top 50 polluters in Canada, as rated by the Trade Publication Corporate Knights, using methods based on those developed by the University.

The AIDS drug Kaletra is made by Abbott Laboratories which the Gates Foundation held 169 million dollars in stock. In 2005, the foundation held nearly 1.5 billion dollars worth of stock in drug companies whose practices have been widely criticized as restricting the flow of key medicines to poor people in developing nations. The Gates Foundation also holds a more than 100 million dollar stake in the vaccine manufacturer Merck.

In 1994, the drug makers, with other research-intensive businesses, lobbied hard and successfully for the international agreement on trade-related aspects of intellectual property rights, which made it harder to move from costly brand name drugs to cheap generics. The agreement protected new-drug monopolies for 20 years or more. Bill Gates and the Gates Foundation activities and funding are key factors in maintaining these intellectual property rights".

Returning to the question of the proliferation of vaccines, we are faced with a broad range of adverse effects including; autism, ADHD, Guillain Barre disease, diabetes, cancer, autoimmune disease, asthma and atopy to name a few. The following is one doctors' testimony presented to a government reform committee hearing on autism in Washington DC April 2000 by Mary Norfleet Megson, MD. Mr. Chairman, Honorable Dan Burton and members of the committee;

"My name is Mary Norfleet Megson.

I am a board-certified pediatrician and a Fellowship Assistant Professor of Pediatrics at the Medical College of Virginia. I have practiced pediatrics for twenty-two years, the last fifteen years seeing only children with Development Disabilities, which include learning disabilities, attention deficit hyperactivity disorder, cerebral palsy, mental retardation and autism.

In 1978, I learned as a resident at Boston Floating Hospital that the incidence of autism was one in 10,000 children. Over the last ten years I have watched the incidence of autism skyrocket to 1/300-1/600 children (the number today is 1/120 children in the US and UK). Over the last nine months, I have treated over 1,200 children in my office. Ninety percent of these children are autistic and from the Richmond area alone. Despite this the State Department of Education reports that there are only 1522 autistic students in the state of Virginia."

Vaccine proponents and most doctors continuously maintain that there is no proof that vaccines are linked to autism despite the exponential increase in autism paralleling the increased usage of vaccines. Despite their apparent certainty, there is a large body of data strongly suggesting that such a linkage exists. The CDC's own investigation corroborates this as was discussed previously.

In the midst of all this controversy it is a clear and unequivocal duty of the medical industry and the medical profession to mandate a definitive study utilizing matched groups of vaccinated and unvaccinated children- to answer this question once and for all. It is clear that there is no intention to do such a study because the almost certain result would be devastating for the vaccine agenda. Such a study would be easy to do and would be definitive and would put an end this decade's long controversy.

It is especially galling that a huge and expensive clinical trial was just completed on 160 thousand women demonstrating that vitamin supplements did not protect from cancer or death (another vitamin study among thousands--Yee Gods!!). Wouldn't it have been far more meaningful to utilize the resources wasted in that study to prove the proposition that vaccines are not linked to autism? Or to save millions more children from becoming autistic?

It might be worthy of note that the vitamin trial failed to make it clear when they reported equal death and cancer rate in both vitamin- takers and non- vitamin takers- that the difference between these two groups represented far more than the attribute of taking a vitamin supplement only. Vitamin-takers universally follow a more healthy life style and are more concerned with factors such as; smoking, drinking, exercise and the healthy life style. Non-vitamin takers tend to eschew the healthy life style for the couch potato life style. Therefore, equivalent cancer and death rate in the two groups, as reported, means either that the healthy life style is of no value or that taking vitamins increases cancer and death rates to the level seen in the smoking and unhealthy like style population. For researchers to ignore the implications of their own studies is a clear expose of the necessity for them to skew their results or suffer boycott by their paymasters.

A landmark study was announced in May 2008, linking vaccine load and autism. The first research project to examine the effects of the "total vaccine load" (at last!) received by children in the 1990's found that autism-like signs and symptoms appeared in infant monkeys vaccinated the same way. The studies principal investigator, Laura Hewitson from the University of Pittsburg, reports developmental delays, behavior problems and brain changes in macaque monkeys that mimic "certain neurological abnormalities of autism." The findings were reported at a major international autism conference in London.

These findings suggest that our closest animal cousins developed characteristics of autism when subjected to the same immunization that American children received when autism diagnoses exploded in the 1990's.

The researchers also reported that "vaccinated animals exhibited progressively severe chronic and active inflammation in gastrointestinal tissue, whereas unexposed animals did not." Numerous scientific studies as well as many parents report severe gastrointestinal ailments in children with regressive autism.

These findings lend credence to studies first published in 1998 by British pediatric gastroenterologist Andrew Wakefield. Wakefield continues to fight against relentless allegations of conflict of interest and improper procedures related to his publication in the Lancet. Of course, perhaps the fact that his paymaster was not a drug company that employs almost all other researchers in this field has something to do with this. Apparently being paid by a drug company is not considered a conflict of interest. As efforts continue to vilify

Andrew Wakefield someone, somewhere, surely must think that if they can somehow discredit this one researcher all the controversy over vaccines and autism will simply evaporate. One would have to wonder why out of all the hundreds of thousands of researchers and research papers Andrew Wakefield is the sole target of questions of conflict of interest?

While the food and drug administration approves individual vaccines as safe and effective, and an advisory committee to the Centers for Disease Control and Prevention recommends the childhood immunization schedule adopted by the states, the overall health outcome from the total vaccine load (now more than 40), versus no vaccination at all, has never been compared.

This rather inexplicable failure necessitated a pending bill in the House of Representatives mandating that the government conduct a study of autism rates in unvaccinated American children.

Former National Institute of Health Director Bernadine Healy called for more research into a possible vaccine link to autism and said, the question had not been settled, despite repeated assertions to that effect by the CDC, the Institute of Medicine and the American Academy of Pediatrics.

It is not within the scope of this book to calculate or disparage the risk/benefit ration of all vaccines, however, a critical look at a few significant examples might show how much more careful we should be of uncritical acceptance of CDC or Institute of Medicine pronouncements.

In the previous chapter the lack of benefit of the seasonal influenza vaccine was rather clearly demonstrated. On top of this, according to the vaccine ADVERSE EVENTS REPORTING SYSTEM (VAERS) the risk of Guillian Barre syndrome (paralysis) increased up to 8 times versus a tetanus - diphtheria vaccine control group. An interesting point about using this particular control group is that the Institute of Medicine itself had concluded that the evidence favors a causal relationship between GBS and tetanus - diphtheria vaccine (the control group used). In interpreting such a study, it should be clearly understood that no more than 10% of vaccine adverse events are ever reported to VAERS.

Prior to reviewing certain specific vaccines I would like to review a number of learned opinions regarding vaccines. The CDC and their experts continue to insist that vaccines are both safe and effective despite considerable evidence to the contrary. In making your own judgment on these issues keep in mind that anyone who claims "certainty" on these issues should be highly suspect. The most telling fact to reiterate ,is that it is totally unconscionable in view of the billions of dollars spent on testing useless "me to" drugs and the endless feckless studies on vitamins and junk science ,no definitive study on the incidence of severe adverse events on vaccinated and unvaccinated US children has been done. This omission is most certainly intentional and is, in my view, a criminal omission by the medical authorities.

Viera Scheibner is a research scientist with a doctorate in natural science. She has published numerous scientific papers and has done extensive research into the relationship between sudden infant death syndrome and vaccines. Her introduction into this issue was through the observation of highly stressed breathing patterns detected by computerized monitoring systems closely related to vaccine administration. She contends that these patterns, juxtaposed with numerous clusters of SIDS death within 21 days of DPT injections, are strong evidence for SIDS deaths being vaccine deaths.

Dr. Scheibner also had this to say regarding vaccines;" no doubt you have heard about the shaken baby syndrome. Only about 10 days ago I was in the United States at a court case testifying about shaken baby syndrome. These are often vaccine deaths. This information was published in NEXUS August -September issue 1998 which resulted in cases of shaken baby syndrome being thrown out of court.

197

The United States is the most developed country in the world with all kinds of money for medical research and advanced medical technology. How is their infant mortality? Before mass vaccination started the United States had the 6th best mortality in the world. By 1990, they were in 20th place. Only a year later they were in the 24th place. Today, maybe 30th place. And most of these deaths are vaccine deaths, so you can camouflage all sorts of things, but you can't lie about infant deaths."

The Japanese Government stopped vaccinating children below the age of 2 years. Sudden infant death cases went from a high 17th place in infant mortality to the lowest infant morality rate in the world.

Health authorities in Australia reveal the vaccination status of children in epidemics. In the last 18 months, 84% of Australian children who got whooping cough were fully vaccinated, and 78% who got measles had a record of measles vaccination. So where is the effectiveness of the vaccine?

William C. Porch, pediatric neurologist published DPT immunization: a potential cause of sudden infant death syndrome in neurology 1982. Of the cases studied 2/3 had been vaccinated within 3 weeks of death.

Following a world wide epidemic of whopping cough 84% of Swedish children who got whooping cough were vaccinated, so the Swedish government discontinued whooping cough vaccination. There is a higher incidence of whooping cough in the first month of life, when infants are most vulnerable, due to the lack of trans- placental immunity from mothers who have been vaccinated.

SIDS AND VACCINES BY HARRIS L. COULTER PHD.
Crib deaths were so infrequent in the pre - vaccination era that it was not even mentioned in the statistics, but it started to

climb in the 1950's with the spread of mass vaccination against diseases of childhood. It became a matter of public and professional concern and acquired a new name, "sudden infant death of unknown origin", or SIDS. We have witnessed a steady rise in the incidence of SIDS, closely following the growth of childhood vaccination, but information on the progress of this epidemic has been radically suppressed in the official literature. Vaccinations of all kinds are now declared absolutely safe at all times and in all places. This has required some fancy footwork with the epidemiologic statistics.

In 1982, matters came to a crisis when William Torch, MD., presented a study to the American Academy of Pediatrics linking the DPT shot with SIDS. Torch's report provoked uproar in the American Academy of Pediatrics. At a hastily arranged press conference he was soundly chastised for using "anecdotal data," meaning "will you believe it?" that he actually interviewed the families concerned!

This mistake was not made again. Gerald M. Fenichel, MD., chairman of the department of neurology at Vanderbilt University Medical Center, in 1983 published an article on vaccinations entitled "The danger of case reports," and the pro-vaccination literature produced in profusion in later years and decades has generally steered away from and around such things as a "case report." God preserve us from contact with the children themselves or their families!"

So the cat was let out of the bag by Dr. Torch, who has been effectively silenced by his colleagues.

A later article on the SIDS - vaccination relationship was published in pediatric infectious diseases January 1983. This found a statistically significant excess of deaths in the first day and the first week after vaccination.

Another study of the SIDS vaccination connection is "DPT immunization and sudden death syndrome" by Alexander

Walker published in the American Journal of Public Health August 1987.

This study found after examining the records of 35 thousand children the SIDS mortality rate in the period 0 to 3 days following the DPT shot to be 7.3 times that in the period beginning 30 days after immunization.

A major campaign was instituted in 1992, to help prevent SIDS by placing babies on their backs. This "back to bed" advice ostensibly reduced SIDS deaths in 2001 by 50%. This result was hailed as proof that SIDS deaths were not related to vaccines.

Certainly this was reassurance to mothers who dutifully presented their babies for an ever- increasing barrage of vaccines. The only problem with all of this was that as the official SIDS death rate declined the overall neonatal death rate went up! According to the national center for health statistics, the US neonatal death rate went from 6.8 per thousand to 7 per thousand. If the SIDS rate, which is the single greatest cause of neonatal death, went down 50% how was it possible for the overall neonatal death rate to go up? If anything, the overall reduction should be greater what would be reflected by the SIDS decrease, because mothers who smoke have double the normal infant death rate and smoking among mothers had dropped precipitously.

Personally, I never gave much credence to the idea that the mothers of SIDS babies were carelessly dumping their babies into their cribs face down, and if they merely had placed them on their backs, they would not have died.

It turns out that this back to bed reduction is simply another statistical dance relating to the international classification of disease revision, which reclassified over half of the SIDS cases into a new category called sudden unexpected infant deaths or SUID. Meanwhile total infant deaths continue to rise and the latest numbers placed the US as

29th in the world, tying us with Slovakia and Poland. This, despite the U.S. spending more on medical costs and neonatal technology than any other country in the world.

I should reiterate here the fact that neither the CDC or any pediatric society, or any doctors have called for, or done, a definitive study comparing vaccinated and unvaccinated children to prove their contention that vaccines are completely safe.

VACCINES AND ALLERGIES

A study in the UK by the department of respiratory medicine at the University of Nottingham in 2002 reported the following:
A follow - up on 29 thousand patients found that patients immunized with the childhood vaccine schedule are 14 times more likely to be diagnosed with asthma and 10 times more likely diagnosed with eczema than unvaccinated children.

In another series of studies in New Zealand, Michel Odent found the frequency of asthma in groups of fully vaccinated children to be between 11% and 23%. In both studies the frequency in the unvaccinated children was only 0 to 1%. Several studies found the rate higher after vaccine that used aluminum hydroxide as adjuvants.

This brings us to an evaluation of one of the latest best selling vaccines for pediatric use. PREVNAR is a vaccine against the organism streptococcus pneumoniae, a common cause of invasive infections in children, including meningitis and pneumonia. PREVNAR happens to contain .125mg of aluminum per .5ml dose!

In the literature accompanying PREVNAR the concentrations of pneumococcal antibodies are listed following the third dose of PREVNAR. It then goes on to state that the minimum serum antibody concentration necessary for protection against invasive pneumococcal disease or against pneumococcal otitis media has not been determined for any serotype.

The literature then lists the following side effects occurring within three days: fever 23%, irritability 52%, drowsiness and restless sleep 54%, decreased appetite 18%, vomiting 13%, diarrhea 10%, rash less than 1%.

To date there have been 416 deaths linked to PREVNAR with or without combination of other vaccines.

With this information in mind it behooves us to examine the purported benefits of PREVNAR, as well as its safety and long term consequences, as a prototype and basis for the chapter to follow on the ever burgeoning list of childhood vaccines.

The following key figures supported and promoted PREVNAR for universal vaccination:

Dr.'s Stephen Black and Henry Shinefield of Kaiser Permanente who undertook the primary studies cited regarding PREVNAR.

Wyeth Lederle, the vaccine's manufacturer, paid for these studies.

These doctors presented PREVNAR at various conferences throughout the world. Wyeth Lederle subsidized these conferences. According to Black "this vaccine is urgently needed... it is great news for parents and physicians." Dr. Shinefield is equally enthusiastic. He states, "It's a remarkable vaccine that will have a dramatic effect."

Wyeth Lederle also pays for an internet forum where Doctors Stephen Pelten and Catherine Edwards address PREVNAR related questions. Wyeth Lederle has paid Dr. Edwards $250.000.per year. Edwards is also one of 15 full time members of the FDA's vaccines and related biological products advisory committee.

Dr. Margaret Rennels was instrumental in getting ROTASHIELD to market and is now involved in PREVNAR. Her university received over $2.5 million from vaccine companies including Wyeth Lederle. She is one of 12 members of the committee on infectious diseases, the committee that makes vaccine recommendations as part of the American Academy of Pediatrics.

Dr. Jerome Kline of Boston Medical Center has enthusiastically called PREVNAR "a big win for kids." Dr. Kline has done his best to protect the financial sanctity of vaccine manufacturers from parents whose children have been injured or killed by a vaccine. He has been hired by the major drug companies to testify in legal cases on behalf of vaccine manufacturers and against vaccine - injured children. Here's one example as summarized from the legal literature:

On August 22, 1984 a healthy nine month old baby named Sean Leary was administered his third DPT vaccine. Sean immediately began vomiting. The next day, he stopped eating. He stayed alert but was no longer active. That night he cried out every 15 to 30 minutes. The pediatrician immediately noted the "obvious circulatory collapse." There at the pediatrician's office, "Sean's eyes rolled back in his head and he stopped breathing." He was rushed to an emergency room. Recitative efforts failed and Sean was pronounced dead at 1:44PM.

Dr. Jerome Kline testified that the relationship between vaccination and Sean's death was "merely coincidental."

Dr. Kline is a member of the National Vaccine Advisory Committee. This committee makes recommendations to the assistant secretary of health concerning vaccine safety and efficacy. He is also the chief editor of Pneumo.com the pro-PREVNAR web site that is "supported by an unrestricted educational grant from Wyeth-Lederle vaccines."

How good is PREVNAR? According to the study paid for by Wyeth Lederle and generated by Dr's Black and Shinefield: "in the primary analysis of all acute otitis media episodes (i.e. earaches), children receiving the investigational pneumococcal vaccine (PREVNAR) had 6% fewer new episodes."

6% fewer episodes of earaches! Do you find that impressive? Keep in mind that there are at least 5 other pediatric vaccines that can cause earaches and ear infection. It appears that we now have PREVNAR, a vaccine designed to prevent adverse effects caused by other vaccines.

What about preventing invasive pneumococcal disease? According to data from the manufacturers insert, after one dose of the vaccine .016% of the recipients (3 out of 18,906) were diagnosed with invasive pneumococcal disease, but, .14% of controls (27 out of 18,910 children who were administered a different experimental vaccine) got invasive pneumococcal disease. Based on this data, PREVNAR decreases a child's chance of getting invasive pneumococcal disease by about 0.1%!

PREVNAR is a bio-engineered product. It is created by combining the protein - polysaccharides from 7 strains of dangerous streptococcus penumoniae bacteria with diphtheria toxin and purified with ammonium sulfate. Such a creation has never before existed and the human race has never before been exposed to such a product.

The insert describes the following: of the 17 thousand subjects who received at least 1 dose of PREVNAR there were 162 visits to the emergency room within 3 days. There were 33 deaths and 13 deaths from SIDS. How do these numbers compare to unvaccinated children? Has there ever been a study to determine this. What about visits to the emergency room or seizures that occurred after the 3 day period? It appears that no such study was completed.

DR. ERDEM CANTEKIN ON THE PNEUMOCOCCAL VACCINE-PREVNAR

Erdem Cantekin PhD. is Professor of Otolaryngology, University of Pittsburg. He is an internationally recognized authority on Otitis media. Dr. Cantekin has published more than a 150 articles in the medical literature. "The alleged benefits for this new vaccine are greatly exaggerated and the risks are significant," said Cantekin. "The bacteria pneumocococcus, with more than 90 serotypes, is a common pathogen. It is not known how pneumocococcus transmutes itself into a pathogen. **The role of pneumocococcus in the micro- biological balance is not known.** The vaccination of newborns with 7 pneumococcal serotypes and possible eradication of those serotypes is an uninformed experiment a best.**" PREVNAR is not effective for otitis media** or pneumonia and the prevention of meningitis data are inconclusive, so why does the American academy of pediatrics want our children to be immunized using PREVNAR?

The big push for PREVNAR came from its supposed prevention of otitis media. The simple fact about otitis media is that 60% of the cases are viral, less than 40% are bacterial and perhaps 25% are due to pneumocococcus. In 2 days, 90% of otitis cases resolve by themselves without treatment.

The FDA data both from Finland and the HMO trials show that the prevention benefit is less that 4%. Despite this, the economic spin goes on.

Pubic health is supposedly in the hands of 3 government agencies; the FDA, the CDC, and the NIH. These 3 pillars of our public health system are more and more in the hands of expert panels and advisory committees. Most experts are in financial relationships with special interest groups and are usually registered with the speaker offices of various manufacturers. In other words they are paid lobbyists.

The danger that Dr. Cantekin is referring to will become clear over the next few pages, but first lets see what PREVNAR has accomplished for our children over the first 7

205

years of its use. A study published in the New England Journal of Medicine 2009 entitled "Effects of Pneumococcal conjugate vaccine on pneumococcal meningitis," had this to say:

Vaccination with pneumococcal vaccine (PREVNAR) decreased the rates of pneumococcal meningitis in children and adults. **However, the incidence of meningitis caused by non - PREVNAR serotypes has increased.**

Let's first look closely at the purported decrease in the meningitis rate. From 1998 to 2005 the incidence of pneumococcal meningitis decreased from 1.13 to 0.79 cases per one hundred thousand persons. At the same time the incidence of non PREVNAR (PCV7) serotype disease increased significantly from .32 to .51 cases per one hundred thousand persons- essentially totally nullifying the decrease in cases produced by PREVNAR use.

Assuming that the reduction from 1.13 to 0.79 was not offset by the increased incidence of non PCV7 serotypes, we see a reduction of 1.13-0.79 or .37 cases per one hundred thousand people. The case fatality rate was 8.4% in children. This means that there were .031 deaths per one hundred thousand persons. **This means that it would be necessary to vaccinate 3.5 million persons to achieve a reduction of 1 death.** One has to look at these numbers several times to be sure of their astounding insignificance!

The sheer absurdity of vaccinating 3.5 million children with a 4 shot regimen at a cost of eight hundred and forty million dollars per year, in order to possibly save one infant life, seems not to occur to the researchers of this study. In truth, this absurdity seems not to occur to anyone in the medical profession. What about the 33 children who died following injection of PREVNAR in the clinical trial? **Even if only of these 33 deaths was caused by PREVNAR that means that we would have to accept 1888 vaccine deaths for the one life saved from meningitis.**

As horrendous as these numbers are, they represent only half of the story:

Since it was shown in the NEJM study that the incidence of non PCV7 serotypes (that is those not covered by PREVNAR) increased and that these organisms were far more resistant to antibiotic treatment the net result certainly must be many more over-all unrecognized deaths.

The response of the researchers to these appalling statistics and to the obvious danger posed by the increase of resistant serotypes was to assure us that further phase 3 clinical trials are underway to evaluate the safety and efficacy of vaccines containing 13 additional serotypes. A 7 serotype containing vaccine is not sufficient for them, they now want to inject infant with 13 vaccines simultaneously.

The article concludes with- what your patients need to know: "tell parents to have their children vaccinated with the pneumococcal vaccine per ACIP recommendations. Patients age 65 or older should receive the 23-valent pneumococcal vaccine"
(PNEUMOVAX 23 -Merck).

It is impossible for me to imagine that these researchers could be looking at the same data that we are looking at and continuing to make these unbelievable recommendations. It is hard for me to avoid the conclusion that such recommendations are a death sentence for thousands of children without concern or liability on the part of those advocating and advising this vaccine.

Reporter Valerie Williams in NEWS 8 INVESTIGATES: PREVNAR- Had this to say (Feb. 2001)
"The vaccine manufacturer of a new vaccine that's added to the universal use list has an assured stable market of 3.5 to 4 million babies born in this country every year. As of 1986 the manufacturer has virtually no liability for adverse events. A stockholders dream.

207

PREVNAR is administered in a series of 4 shots, each priced about $60.00. It one of the most expensive vaccines in history.

Hayley Graves was 9 months old when she received her 2nd dose of PREVNAR "I had a baby that was perfectly healthy, happy, ok until she got a shot, until she got her vaccine," said her father, Ray Graves. "30 hours later, she is in the hospital having seizures that they can't stop. Hayley slipped in and out of a coma for 45 days until she died in September. Tremors shook her little body almost the entire time."

Like many parents, Ray and Lisa Graves were told by their pediatrician that PREVNAR would help to prevent otitis media (ear infection).

NEWS 8 discovered that PREVNAR was never licensed for that use. In fact, clinical trials showed that PREVNAR decreased a child's chance of getting an ear infection by only 6%.

Dr. Erdem Cantekin, a medical researcher, is one of the nations leading experts on ear infection. "PREVNAR is an ineffective and toxic vaccine, "he said.

Cantekin says a study by the vaccine manufacturer shows seizures happen 4 times more often in infants given vaccines with PREVNAR than children in a control group.

Before licensing PREVNAR last year, vaccine committees from both the FDA and the CDC dismissed the data on seizures as insignificant. However, as part of our investigation, NEWS 8 reviewed nearly 800 adverse reactions reports filed with the FDA during the past 9 months. We found that one out of 10 children who had side effects suffered some sort of seizure."

The following article appearing in April 2008, by Health editor Jeremy Laurence, brings to the fore-front one of the most serious long term and deleterious effects caused by vaccines, and almost totally ignored:

INCREASE IN SEVERE PNEUMONIA IN CHILDREN MAY BE CAUSED BY VACCINE.

Cases of a life threatening pneumonia that affects the young are rising rapidly in Britain. It now affects around 1000 children a year. The cause of the increase is unknown, but experts fear a vaccine in the immunization program could be contributing.

Child health specialists say cases of the pneumonia, known as serotype 1, have risen 10-fold in a decade. They warned that a vaccine against pneumococcal disease called PREVNAR introduced in 2006 could be fueling the rise.
There are more than 90 known strains of the bacterium that causes pneumonia. When one is eliminated, it creates an opportunity for another to take its place. In the US, where PREVNAR was introduced in 2000, researchers have reported an emergence of "sero-replacement" disease types of pneumonia not covered by the vaccine.

NON-PCV7 PNEUMOCOCCAL DISEASE INCREASING IN SPAIN
The introduction of 7-valent pneumococcal conjugate vaccine (PCV7) in Spain in 2001 has been followed by the emergence of invasive pneumococcal disease caused by virulent disease clones of non-PCV7 serotypes.

In the January 15 issue of Clinical Infectious Diseases, Dr. Carmen Munoz-Almagro of the University of Barcelona and colleagues report their study of the incidence of culture-proven invasive pneumococcal disease.

"The post PREVNAR period, in children aged less than 5 years, has shown an increase in the rate of pneumonia and empyema of 320% caused by non-PCV7 serotypes.

A review by Lipsitch in the CDC's Emerging Infectious Diseases Perspectives detailed pneumococcal serotype replacement in several studies and concluded "the occurrence of serotype replacement in 3 trials of pneumococcal conjugant

209

vaccines confirmed the validity of concerns expressed in anticipation of these trials."

Doctors and clinics pay $69.25 for each of the 4 required doses of PREVNAR, amounting to approximately 40% of the total cost of recommended pediatric vaccines. The financial performance of the vaccine has been remarkable, amounting to net revenue in 2005 of more than 1.6 billion dollars. During 2005 PREVNAR was launched in 13 additional international markets. At the same time, in 2005, researchers from the CDC disclosed the following results in the Journal of Infectious Diseases, December 2005:
The introduction of the 7-valant pneumococcal vaccine (PCV7) in children has resulted in serotype replacement. The rate of serotype replacement in children less than 5 years old increased significantly from 2.6 cases per one hundred thousand population to 6.5 cases per hundred thousand population.
 This was accompanied by significant increases in penicillin non susceptibility and multi- drug resistance.

There were 3 more extremely disturbing studies published in April of 2006.
CLINICAL INFECTIOUS DISEASES APRIL 2006:
Emergence of vaccine-related pneumococcal serotypes as a cause of bacteremia. This study concluded that rates of penicillin resistant bacteremia (septicemia) increased significantly due to vaccine-related serotypes.
PEDIATRIC INFECTIOUS JOURNAL 2006
Changing epidemiology of outpatient bacteremia in children after the introduction of conjugated pneumococcal vaccine.
"In the United States as the incidence of pneumococcal bacteremia has decreased, E. coli, salmonella, and staphylococcus aureus have increased in relative importance"
NEW ENGLAND JOURNAL OF MEDICINE APRIL 2006

210

Effect of introduction of the pneumococcal conjugate vaccine on drug resistant streptococcus pneumonia.

While rates of all resistant diseases caused by the vaccines serotypes fell 87%, rates of serotype 19A-related disease, a deadly type in the very young, rose by 315%. And while rates of multiple drug resistant pneumococcal infections peaked at 4.1 cases per hundred thousand in 1999, rates of serotype 19A - related disease in children peaked at a remarkable 8.3 cases per one hundred thousand in 2004.

Lastly, they stated, that in addition to serotype 19A, there are some 80 serotypes of pneumococcus that are not included in the vaccine, each with its own cadre of troubles.

It is clear that were are in the process of replacing strains of pneumococcus with more virulent and antibiotic resistant organisms that will kill far more than we can possibly help with this vaccine. We are playing an ecological form of Russian roulette. It would appear that this reality is being overridden world-wide by the rampaging financial success of this vaccine.

Researchers have estimated that there are now 90 thousand deaths per year due to antibiotic resistant organisms (MRSA'S) caused by the combined effect of antibiotic overuse and vaccines.

In 2005, there were reported to VAERS 416 childhood deaths after PREVNAR plus other vaccine administration and 11 deaths associated with PREVNAR alone. (Keep in mind VAERS reports are not mandatory and constitute less than 10% of actual cases).

The previously noted New England Journal of Medicine article proved that 3.5 million children must be given the 4 dose regimen of PREVNAR containing 7 serotypes, for an essential total of 28 vaccines, in order to prevent a single death from meningitis. Counter balancing this single death against

211

the hundreds of vaccine deaths and possible thousands of MRSA deaths (resistant organisms) caused by this vaccine it is completely unexplainable how virtually every pediatrician continues to advise parents to subject their babies to this vaccine.

So now that you have been given this background information as to how egregious the vaccine agenda can be, it will be useful to scan through a few more of the miracle vaccines of the 21 century.

CHAPTER XVIII
OUR CUP RUNNETH OVER

We will now examine a selection of vaccines that your doctor will be recommending for your child with absolute assurances of, safe, very safe - of course it's safe.

An article in Natural News by Mike Adams is entitled The Great HPV (human papilloma virus) - Gardasil:

For the past several years HPV vaccines have been marketed to the public and mandated in compulsory injections for young girls in several states, based on the idea that they prevent cervical cancer. Now, Natural News has obtained documents from the FDA and other sources which reveal that the FDA has been well aware for several years that human papilloma virus (HPV) has no direct link to cervical cancer.
Natural News has also learned that HPV vaccines have been proven to be flatly worthless in clearing the HPV virus from women who have already been exposed to HPV (which includes most sexually active women), calling into question the scientific justification of mandatory "vaccinate everyone" policies.

Furthermore, this story reveals evidence that the vaccine currently being administrated for HPV - Gardasil- may increase the risk of precancerous cervical lesions by an alarming 44.6% in some women. The vaccine, it turns out, may be far more dangerous to the health of women than doing nothing at all.

If true, this information reveals details of an enormous public health fraud being perpetrated on American people, involving FDA officials, big Pharma promoters, and even the governors of states like Texas. The health and safety of tens of millions of young girls is at stake here, and what this Natural News investigative report reveals is that HPV vaccination may not only be medically useless it may also be harmful to the health of the young girls receiving them.

This report also revealed that the FDA has, for 4 years, known that HPV was not the cause of cervical cancer and that HPV infections are self-limiting and pose no real danger to healthy women.

In the course of documenting a petition to the FDA by the manufacturers of a DNA testing device that can detect the presence of HPV the following information was revealed: An FDA news release of 2003 acknowledges that "most infections by HPV are short-lived and not associated with cervical cancer. Most women who become infected with HPV are able to eradicate the virus and suffer no apparent long term consequences to their health."

Based on new scientific information published in the last 15 years, it is now generally agreed that identifying and typing HPV infection does not bear a direct relationship to the risk of cervical cancer. Most acute infections caused by HPV are self-limiting. Repeated sequential transient HPV infections, even when caused by high risk HPV's are characteristically not associated with high risk of developing precursor lesions of cervical cancer. It is persistent infection, not the virus that determines the cancer risk.

Vaccination with Gardasil of women who are already sero-positive and PCR-positive for vaccine-relevant HPV has been found to increase the risk of developing high grade pre-cancerous lesions by 44.6% according to an FDA VRBPAC background document : Gardasil HPV quadrivalent, May 18,2006 VRBPAC meeting.

There were 2 important concerns that were identified during the course of this efficacy review. One was the potential for Gardasil to enhance disease among a sub-group who had evidence of persistent infection with vaccine relevant HPV types. The other concern was the observation of the potential for HPV types not contained in the vaccine to counter the efficacy of Gardasil on HPV types contained in the vaccine. **In other words the vaccine, if given to a young woman who already carries HPV in a harmless state, may**

215

activate the infection and directly cause precancerous lesions to appear.

Research published in the Journal of the American Medical Association August 2007, entitled" Effect of Human Papilloma Virus vaccine among young women with preexisting infection," (this includes virtually all women for a sexually active, regardless of their age) reached the following conclusion, **"no significant evidence of a vaccine therapeutic effect was observed** in analyses restricted to women who received all doses of vaccine or those with evidence of single HPV infection at entry. Similarly, no evidence of vaccine effects was observed in analyses stratified by other study entry parameters."

In other words, the authors found no evidence that the vaccine worked at all. This observation led the authors to offer a final conclusion: "rates of viral clearance over a 12 month period are not influenced by vaccination. Given that viral clearance rates did not differ by treatment group and that persistent viral infection is the best established predictor of risk of progression, it is unlikely that vaccination could have a significant beneficial impact on rate of lesion progression."

Natural News believes Merck is currently engaged in a massive medical fraud, and that it has influenced, corrupted or otherwise recruited FDA officials and state health authorities in a grand scheme that is at best medically worthless, and at worst medically dangerous. Halting cervical cancer seems to have nothing to do with the marketing and prescribing of Gardasil. The entire campaign push for mandatory HPV vaccinations seems to be based entirely in the realm of sales and marketing. "

It is beyond doubt that vaccination with Gardasil has not been proven to prevent a single case of cervical cancer. However, the latest Gardasil statistics reported to the FDA include 9000 adverse reactions (including paralysis) and 27 deaths between 2006 and 2008.

U.S. cancer statistics show that there are 30 to 40 cervical cancer cases per one million women per year between the ages of 9 and 26, which is the age bracket that Gardasil targets and was tested on. According to Merck, Gardasil was shown to reduce pre-cancers by 12.2% to 16.5% in the general population. So instead of ending up with 30 to 40 cases of cancer per million per year, in that age bracket, the HPV vaccine can potentially bring it down to 26 to 35 cases of cervical cancer.

What that means is that you would have to vaccinate one million girls to prevent cancer in 4.

Further, about 37% of women who develop cervical cancer actually die from the disease so **vaccinating one million girls would prevent 1 death per year** at a price of 360 million dollars per year. [Assuming Gardasil works at all]

As previously stated between 2006 and 2008 there have already been 27 deaths due to vaccination with Gardasil as well as life threatening ailments, spontaneous abortions and birth defects.

The current treatment of precancerous lesions has limited the progression to actual cancer to only 1%. Use of a now suppressed antiviral vaginal gel would most certainly reduce this 1% significantly. (Read- ALPHAMIR vaginal gel) Therefore, in view of the previously presented data and the fact that there are more than one hundred types of human papilloma virus, of which Gardasil potentially reduces only 4 , any possible or apparent usefulness of this vaccine becomes a virtual impossibility. Moreover, if you have already been exposed to one of the 4 types of virus that is in the vaccine, it increases your risk of cervical cancer.

Gardasil has caused a number of deaths due to blood clots, acute respiratory failure, cardiac arrest, and sudden death of unknown cause, shortly after its administration. Other reported side effects include spontaneous abortions, genital

217

warts, anaphylactic shock, seizures, coma and paralysis. 5 subjects that got the vaccine had babies with birth defects whereas no birth defects occurred among the subjects who received the placebo. In the past year there were a total of 1637 reported adverse effects.

Drug companies are immune from prosecution for these deaths and adverse events, however, US tax-payers foot the bill of the more than 1.5 billion dollars which has been paid out by the US Government.

As if to put a final closure on this saga of Gardasil, a recent study in the Journal of the American Medical Association states that the rates for HPV 16 and 18 - the two types purported to be responsible for most cervical cancers- are astronomically low: only 1.5% and .08% respectfully, and even among those cases 90% disappear on their own.

Just as we saw the continued advocation of the use of PREVNAR despite overwhelming data against its use, we again see continued advocation of the use of Gardasil by medical doctors entrusted with the care of your children, despite the overwhelming evidence against it.

It would appear that it now becomes the responsibility of parents to prevent their children from receiving ineffective and unsafe vaccines so glibly advocated by senior health officials and pediatricians.

Next-- ROTAVIRUS: DEATH BY DIARRHEA? An article from Inside Vaccines regarding ROTASHIELD and ROTATEQ vaccines, February 2008.

"Rotavirus is reported to be the leading cause of diarrhea among children, causing upwards of 55 thousand hospitalizations per year in the US. The first rotavirus vaccine (ROTASHIELD) was recalled in 1999, for causing intussusception, which is a serious and life threatening condition where the intestine becomes obstructed.

In 2006, a new rotavirus vaccine (ROTATEQ) was approved by the FDA. My family doctor strongly recommended the new vaccine. Each year an estimated 54 thousand US children are hospitalized for diarrhea, but less than 12 die with rotavirus. Since there are approximately 1/5 the number of deaths from rotavirus in the population then occurs from lightning strikes, the question must be asked why such a vaccine is necessary.

The answer, I am afraid, was contained in an article from the Journal of Pediatrics 2004 on use of rotavirus vaccine in healthy infants. At the conclusion of the article we find the following: Dr's. H. Fred Clark, David I. Bernstein, Penelope H. Dennehy, Paul Offit, Michael Picherero, John Treanor and Richard L. Ward received funding for research or for clinical investigation from Merck and Company Inc.
Dr's Clark and Offit are co- holders of a patent on rotavirus vaccine. Dr. Dennehy also is a member of the Merck speaker's bureau. Dr's David L. Krah, Allan Shaw, Michael Dallas, Karen Kaplan and Penny Heaton are current employees and Dr's Joseph Eiden and Natalie Ivanoff are former employees of Merck and Company Inc.
Patent holder Dr. Paul Offit was a member of the CDC's advisory committee of Immunization Practices.

Somewhere in the above exposition one might find the answer to why we need ROTATEQ.

Documents from the CDC show that 95% of children have had rotavirus by age 5 and that after one natural infection 88% of children are protected against severe diarrhea.

As for treatment, even the CDC believes that acute gastroenteritis can be properly cared for at home. "Treatment with ORS (oral rehydration solutions such as pediolyte) is simple and enables management of uncomplicated cases of diarrhea at home, regardless of the etiologic agent."

About 12 deaths occur each year due to rotavirus diarrhea among children younger than 5 years. This is a cumulative incidence by age 5 of 0.000004.

As of August 2008, there have been 10,500 reports of adverse events following ROTATEQ vaccine injection, **including 28 deaths.** There were also 375 cases of intussusception. It has been claimed that this is not more than would be expected. That conclusion is based on VAERS reports which we know are never more than 10% of the actual adverse events and upon a study which cited only intussusceptions which occurred within 7 days of injection.

Since the death rate without vaccine is 12 per year and since ROTATEQ does not effectively protect all vaccinated children, in the best of circumstances, no more than 6 to 8 deaths per year could be prevented-- requiring the vaccination of 3.5 million children.
This is certainly no more than would be caused by the vaccine alone, resulting in a net benefit of zero. Moreover, as we have seen with prior vaccines, vaccine use invariably creates an ecological hole filled by more virulent organisms resulting in an increased overall death rate.

One out of 1300 children given ROTATEQ suffered seizures which could lead to severe long term disability. The cumulative death and disability related to the use of this vaccine simply cannot possibly be off-set by the 1.7 deaths per million children vaccinated per year that could be prevented by its use.

Again, one has to look at these figures over and over to appreciate how small the possible benefit can be and to realize how poorly we are being served by the advocates of these vaccines.

While we are being told how safe these vaccines are, the US. Government is secretly and quietly paying billions of dollars in compensation to their victims.

MENACTRA AND "THE HEART BREAK OF MENINGITIS"

It is impossible to conclude that the entire medical industry is so universally and incredibly stupid as to put evermore dangerous and useless drugs and vaccines into our prescriptions and into the bodies of our children.

It becomes a semantic exercise as to what constitutes criminal negligence versus manslaughter, or even murder. For reasons almost inexplicable to me - the persons behind these felonious activities seem unconcerned about the possible unraveling of the cover-up, which might lead to some level of accountability. On the contrary, they seem to move inexorably from bad to worse as we have seen in our journey through the data.

If these words seem overly harsh, take another journey with me through the story of the new "life saving" vaccine MENACTRA.

A journey yet another step deeper into the rat hole. A salient fact about these vaccines is that most parents are totally unaware of their mandated and ever- increasing application to their children. Ask any parent if they have heard of PREVNAR or MENACTRA and you will receive a silent stare.   If parents are unaware of what vaccines their children are getting - how many do you think have an inkling about the data that describes their validity?

MENACTRA is a vaccine to save us and our children from the dread disease "meningococcal meningitis", a rare form of meningitis caused by the organism Neisseria Meningitidis.

Tipping the scales away from ignorance and toward deliberate deception is the carefully orchestrated "fear mongering" theatrical program which accompanies the promotional efforts for MENACTRA.

Bereaved families of meningitis victims are trotted out as long suffering stalwart soldiers in the fight against the horror of meningitis - "if we could save just one life - it will be worth it".

On the manufacturers web site (SANOFI- PASTEUR) we are shown a gaggle of vibrant young children and admonished that we must keep their dreams alive with a shot of MENACTRA. This same web site also solicits stories from persons who have had personal experience with meningococcal disease, to be used for promotional purposes.

Promotions as in the following story from MSNBC Health News:

KILLER AT COLLEGE: MENINGITIS THREATENS STUDENTS

When Lynn Bozof's son Evan was a teenager there was a meningitis outbreak in a neighboring county. Evan was worried, and he asked his mom if he should get the vaccination. She remembers her reply "oh Evan, you don't need to worry about meningitis!"

But five years later, at a Georgia Southwestern University in 1988, Evan called his mom complaining of a migraine. It got so bad that he went to the emergency where he was diagnosed with meningitis and placed in intensive care. His kidneys shut down. His liver stopped functioning. Both arms and legs had to be amputated. After a 26 day fight against the disease, Evan died.

As Lynn Bozof watched her son's losing battle, a memory of a teenage Evan asking about meningitis cruelly replayed in her mind. "I feel like that came back to haunt me because I didn't take the time to find out about the disease," she says. "Just because this disease is rare doesn't mean it is not going to affect you or someone you know."

This and other heart rending stories are repeated over and over, as in the case of Ashley. In Ashley's case the doctors at first assumed she was merely dehydrated and tried to send her home, the family remembers. Even after a purplish rash - a classic sign of meningitis - spread over her body, emergency room staff still had no idea what was wrong.

Terrified for his daughter, Ashley's dad, Tom, demanded that she be transferred to a larger hospital. Ashley screamed in pain the entire time it took the ambulance to get to the hospital in Indianapolis, 77 miles away. "It was a ride from hell," Ashley recalled.

As Ashley fought for her life in the hospital, she and her father made the devastating decision to let her doctors take her left foot and three of her fingers.

Ashley spent the last summer covering up the lasting marks of meningitis. The following year when she returned to school, she made a series of bold moves: she put on a tank top, she had her seven remaining singers professionally manicured, and she started to tell her story.

She feels as if it is her responsibility to educate people about the devastating effect of meningitis and to urge others to get the vaccine. She works closely with the National Meningitis Association and has appeared in an informational video the non -profit group produced. On campus, where she is majoring in biology in hopes of going to medical school, she plays the video and speaks to classes about her experience. And she's fielded technical questions about her condition from crowds of doctors and researchers.

She and her family still get angry at times, thinking about the vaccination that she nearly received. The vaccination that could have prevented all this.

But telling her story over and over again can be draining for Ashley. She has to relive the pain, the ambulance ride, the surgeries and every detail of her nightmarish experience yet again. But it's worth it, she says, "even if I can save just one person."

I could add many other such heart rending promotional stories designed to scare , including an NBC News video where Dr. Nancy Snyderman tells us how we can prevent this disease and shares the tragic story of Mackenzie Hartwig ,(Today Show Health) however, I'm sure you have get the picture by now, and I will spare you.

Certainly these stories are unsettling; however, I find them far less troubling than the anguish facing a parent whose child dies following an elective vaccine injection. What can console them?

Not withstanding the theatrics just shown or the oft repeated MENACTRA mantra "if we can save just one life - it would be worth it," dare we examine the reality that lies in the data? I don't think anybody wants us to do that - in fact - I'm pretty sure they doubt that anybody will. But, we are going to do it anyway.

Both the CDC and the Canadian Public Health Service put the case rate of meningococcal disease at approximately 0.9 cases per one hundred thousand population. This number appears to be considerably higher than more recent figures published in the Pediatric Infectious Disease Journal of March 2009. That study followed the results of the Universal Canadian Childhood Vaccination Program.

By 2005, all Canadian Provinces included meningitis strain C vaccine as part of routine childhood vaccination.

"There was a dramatic decline in provinces with the early immunization program, suggesting the program works," says, Dr. Julie Bettinger, a scientist in the vaccine evaluation center at the University of British Columbia. (Note use of the word" suggesting").

Prior to meningitis C vaccination Alberta and Quebec Provinces had rates of meningococcal disease nearly 4.5 times higher than the rest of Canada. Following the vaccination program the rates in these provinces went from 0.41 cases per one hundred thousand people in 2002 down to 0.07 per one hundred thousand in 2006. **The provinces with later introduction showed no major changes in the one year of follow up study,** with annual rates at 0.08 per one hundred thousand people in 2006.

"The numbers may seem small, but even one case of the disease is one to many," says Dr. Bettinger. (Paraphrasing the mantra).

No change in the later provinces! Could it be that the decline in Quebec had nothing to do with the vaccine, but was a natural leveling off to the same rate seen in all other provinces? How is it possible for a vaccine to work in 2 provinces with no effect anywhere else? And did Dr. Bettinger not take notice of this anomaly?

According to this study the incidence of meningitis C throughout Canada is .08 cases per one hundred thousand population. Since the C strain is responsible for 50% of cases, the incidence for all serotypes would be double, or approximately .18 cases per hundred thousand people. How does this reconcile with the CDC and the Canadian Health number of 0.9 cases per hundred thousand?

No one is asking that question, and I must admit that I don't know the answer. So I am going to split the difference between the two and assume a figure half way between them to be as close as can be ascertained. Therefore, midway between 0.9 and 0.18 is 0.5 cases per hundred thousand.

Assuming a case rate of .5 per hundred thousand and utilizing the Canadian death rate statistic of 6.9% we can calculate that there are .035 deaths per hundred thousand population from meningococcal disease.

The CDC has advised that MANACTRA be given to people between the ages of 11 to 55 and seek to mandate more than 40 million people to be injected with MANACTRA. 40 million injections will cost 8 billion dollars and this may have to be followed up by a booster dose at some point, as yet not determined.

Since the vaccine does not protect against type B meningitis which causes 50% of the cases, and since the vaccine is only 50% effective on the strains that are in the vaccine, the maximum theoretical effectiveness is 25%- that is 50% of 50%. Assuming Menactra could save 25% of the death total- 25% of .035 deaths per hundred thousand is .00875 deaths prevented per hundred thousand persons vaccinated. Put in another way, it would be necessary to vaccinate 11.4 million people to save 1 life from meningitis. (Not to mention a cost of 2.3 billion dollars).

No wonder the oft repeated mantra is, "if we could just save one life it would be worth it." Therefore, if the targeted number of 40 million persons were to be reached there would be a theoretical saving of 4 lives - or would there?

Just how much suffering and deaths would the saving of these 4 lives engender? If we look at the VAERS reports on MENATCRA as of November 2008 involving nearly 4 million vaccinations we can extrapolate the toll of 40 million vaccinations by multiplying by 10. These are the numbers. Keep in mind that the VAERS reports are less than 10% of the true figure.

Total reports: 44 thousand
Life threatening reports: 575
Emergency room visits: 16,667
Did not recover: 3,930
Deaths: 60
Lupus: 60
Multiple sclerosis: 70
Paralysis: 260
Rheumatoid arthritis: 60
Seizures: 1,580

Not to mention the following adverse reactions:
Local pain and swelling 59%
Headache 35%
Fatigue 30%
Aching joints 17%

Diarrhea 12%
Loss of appetite 10%
Chills and fever 5%
Vomiting 2%

In addition to all this, a vaccine safety report issued by the NVIC found a huge increased risk of reports of Guillian-Barre paralysis when MANACTRA and Gardasil were administered simultaneously.

And finally, the always ignored problem of serotype replacement by more virulent and resistant strains must be considered, even though the true number of deaths from this phenomenon is as yet unknown.

In my humble opinion, these numbers are an indictment of the entire medical establishment, and I will leave it to your judgment whether they represent criminal behavior or are a combination of greed, avarice, arrogance and sheer stupidity. The next subject may help.

THE HEPATITIS B VACCINE   this one will take us to the furthest reaches of the rat hole.

First, a story from Michael Belkin told in congressional testimony:

"My daughter Lyla Rose Belkin died on September 16, 1998 at the age of 5 weeks, shortly after receiving a hepatitis B vaccine booster shot. The following comments are intended to be a heads up to parents and potential parents about the risks of the hepatitis vaccine, and a first hand report questioning the scientific legitimacy of the vaccine industry, which provides eight hundred million dollars of annual revenue to Merck - the company which makes the hepatitis vaccine distributed in the US.

Lyla Rose Belkin was a lively, alert 5 week old baby when I last held her in my arms. Little did I imagine, as she gazed intently into my eyes with all the innocence and wonder of a new born child, that she would die that night. She was never ill before receiving the hepatitis shot that afternoon. At her final feeding that night, she was agitated and feisty - and then fell asleep and didn't wake up. The autopsy ruled out choking. A swollen brain was the only abnormal finding. Most doctors I spoke to at the time said it must have been sudden infant death syndrome.

The first instinctive reaction in such a situation is for parents to blame themselves. The logical part of my brain kept returning to the obvious medical event that preceded Lyla's death - and that internal voice kept asking the question, could the hepatitis vaccine that Lyla received that afternoon have killed her? Most doctors I asked scoffed at that notion and said the vaccine was perfectly safe. But I began to search around on the internet and med line and discovered disturbing evidence of adverse reactions to this vaccine.

In the US. Hepatitis B disease mainly infects intravenous drug users, homosexuals, prostitutes and promiscuous heterosexuals. The disease is transmitted by blood, through sex or dirty needles. How could a newborn baby possibly get hepatitis B if the mother was screened and tested negative as my wife was? So why are most US babies inoculated at birth by their hospital or pediatrician with hepatitis B vaccine?

I have discovered that the answer is; an unrestrained health bureaucracy decided it couldn't get junkies, gays, prostitutes and promiscuous heterosexuals to take the vaccine, so they mandated that all babies must be vaccinated at birth. Drug companies such as Merck (reaching for new markets) were instrumental in pushing government scientists to adopt and at-birth hepatitis B vaccination policy; although the vaccine was never tested in newborns and no vaccine had ever been mandated at birth before.

My search for answers about a link between the hepatitis B vaccine and my daughter's death led me to a hepatitis B vaccine workshop on October 26 at the National Academy of Scientists Institute of Medicine, entitled Vaccine safety forum - neonatal deaths. The NAS was concerned enough about reports of hepatitis B vaccine- related infant deaths and adverse reactions to hold a special workshop on the subject. Dr's and scientists flew in from all over the US and Europe to attend. I sat back and soaked it all up. It was a real eye opener.

The presentation included a study of animal models of newborn response to antigen presentation which showed that newborn immune systems were undeveloped and strikingly different than those of adults.
Another presentation by vaccine researcher Dr Bonnie Dunbar of Baylor Collage related numerous hepatitis B vaccine related cases of nervous system damage in adults, such as multiple sclerosis, seizures and blindness.
 The FDA presented a seemingly reassuring study from its vaccine adverse events reporting system (VAERS) which showed only 19 neonatal deaths reported since 1991 related to hepatitis B vaccine.

I found the VAERS study data to be completely deceptive. I was sitting in that room and my daughter had died during their sample period and wasn't counted. In fact, the New York City coroner called VAERS to report my daughter's death and no one ever returned their call! What kind of reporting system doesn't return the call of the New York City medical examiner - and how many other reports were ignored?

To conclude that the hepatitis B vaccine is safe because VAERS only reports 19 deaths is scientific fraud. In fact I obtained the raw data from the VAERS system and found 54 reported SIDS cases after hepatitis B vaccination in just the 18 months from January 1996 to May 1997. That's almost 15

229

times as many deaths per year as their own flawed study reported. There are seventeen thousand reports of adverse reaction to hepatitis B vaccine in the 1996 - 1997 raw data which the CDC dismisses as a coincidence.

This vaccine has no benefit what-so-ever for newborns, in fact it wears off and they will need booster shots later in life when they actually could be exposed to the disease. This is simply a case of ravenous corporate greed and mindless bureaucracy teeming up to overwhelm common sense. Merck in particular, has gone over the edge with this vaccination program, ignoring and suppressing reports of adverse reactions to their profitable hepatitis B vaccine, which verges on criminal conduct."

TESTIMONY BEFORE THE COMMITTEE ON IMMUNIZATION PRACTICES - CDC, FEBRUARY 1999 by Michael Belkin, former quantitative strategist at Salomon Brothers and director of the hepatitis B vaccine project of the national vaccine information center (NVIC).

"The NVIC has studied VAERS data obtained under the freedom information act covering the last 9 years on hepatitis B vaccine adverse events - and in 1996 there were more than 3 times as many reported serious adverse reactions as reported cases of the disease in the 0 to 14 age group. Of the total 2424 adverse event reports in children under age 14 who only received hepatitis B vaccine, there were 1209 serious events and 73 deaths.

A benefit/risk analysis of the hepatitis B vaccine must conclude that the VAERS data on adverse reactions shows the real-world risk of a newborn infant dying or being injured by the hepatitis B vaccine is a greater threat than the remote chance of contracting the primarily blood transmitted disease.

At NVIC, we are overwhelmed following up constant new reports of death, seizures and autoimmune reactions following hepatitis B vaccination. Because the CDC refuses to acknowledge this large number of serious adverse reactions, hospitals and doctors who have been misled about the risks, continue to administer the vaccine and then deny any vaccine connection when children die, get ill or have seizures within hours or days. CDC officials tell parents they have never heard of hepatitis B vaccine reactions. That is a lie. For this government to continue to insist that hepatitis B vaccine adverse reaction reports do not exist is negligent, unethical - and is a crime against the children of America.

Question: what are the risks and benefits for administering this vaccine to infants?

Answer: hepatitis B is a rare, mainly blood transmitted disease. In 1996 only 54 cases of the disease were reported to the CDC in the 0 to 1 age group. There were 3.9 million births, so the observed incidence of hepatitis B was 0.001% .In the VAERS reporting system there were 1080 total reports of adverse reactions in 1996 in the 0 to 1 age group with 47 deaths reported. (The death rate from hepatitis B is less than 0.1%). Total VAERS hepatitis B adverse reports for the 0-1 age group out-number reported cases of the disease 20 to 1.

The total of 24,775 VAERS hepatitis B reports from July 1990 to October 1998 show 439 deaths and 9673 severe reactions involving emergency room visits, hospitalization, disablement or death."

The National Vaccine Information Center maintains that Federal and State Public Health Officials are promoting forced vaccinations with hepatitis B vaccine without truthfully informing the public about the risks of hepatitis B disease in

America or the known and unknown risk of hepatitis B vaccine.

Unlike other infectious diseases for which vaccines have been developed and mandated in the US, hepatitis B is not common in childhood and is not highly contagious. Hepatitis B is primarily an adult disease transmitted through infected body fluids or dirty needles.

In cases of acute hepatitis B most patients do not require hospital care and 95% of patients have a favorable course and recover completely. The case fatality rate is very low-- less than 0.1 %,(a figure which would be significantly reduced with the utilization of available anti-viral technology).

Those who recover completely from hepatitis B infection acquire life-long immunity (95%). Of the 5% who do not recover completely, fewer than 5% of those become chronic carriers of the disease, and just 1/4 of these are in danger of developing life threatening liver disease later in life.

The purported rationale given by the "experts" for the use of this vaccine is to prevent deaths from liver cancer secondary to chronic hepatitis B infection. One can hardly overstate the absurdity of this preposterous concern. We have already seen the numbers, 95% of cases of hepatitis B infection recover completely. 0.0625% of those who get hepatitis B end up having liver disease when they reach the age of 60 or more. Put in another way, 1 in 2000 drug addicts who contract hepatitis B will die of liver cancer, between 50 and 80 years of age, if they don't die first of a drug overdose.

In the year 2007 there were a total of 16,000 cases of liver cancer in the United States: of these 95% were secondary to alcoholism. Of the remaining 800 cases of liver cancer from all causes only, at most, 1 to 2 hundred could be attributed to hepatitis B infection. **And not one of these liver cancers would have been prevented by a hepatitis B vaccination at birth. The entire purported rationale is an obvious and total fraud-- by the time these people contracted hepatitis**

B infection, the efficacy of a vaccine given at birth would have long since worn off.

Fifteen thousand French citizens filed a law suit against the French Government for understating the risk and overstating the benefits associated with hepatitis B vaccine. Hundreds of people were reported to have suffered from autoimmune and neurological disorders, including multiple sclerosis, following hepatitis B vaccination. As a result, in October 1998, the French Minister of Health ended the mandatory hepatitis B vaccination program for all school children. This was followed up by--

AN ENLIGHTENING LETTER TO THE WORLD HEALTH ORGANIZATION
This letter was sent to Dr. Jong-Wook Lee, Director General of the World Health Organization on 17 November 2005 by Dr. Marc Girard.

Dear. Dr. Lee,
Further to the universal campaign against hepatitis B launched in France in September 1994 upon the recommendations of the WHO, a criminal inquiry has been opened on demand of the relatives of people, some of them children, who died after being immunized; having been commissioned as a medical expert witness by the French Judge, I have spent thousands of hours on this subject, and had access to dozens of confidential documents.

Although my reports are still secret by court order, a number of my findings were leaked after being transmitted to the litigants; in addition, the arrogance and impunity of the experts involved has been such that it is possible to find a significant echo of my observations in published data.

In February 2004, I read a correspondence by an Indian colleague, Dr. J. Puliyel (Lancet 2004) on the fallacies of the data spread by the WHO about the epidemiology of hepatitis B in his country. I was struck by the fact that the mechanism of the deception as described by Dr. Puliyel (gross exaggeration, lack of references, inappropriate extrapolations..) were exactly comparable to those I observed in my own country - and of course with the same results; a plea of "experts" to include hepatitis B vaccination in the National Vaccination Program, in spite of its cost and, I may add, of its unprecedented toxicity.

It is blatant that in the promotion of the hepatitis B vaccination, the WHO has never been more than a screen for an undue commercial promotion, in particular via the Viral Hepatitis Prevention Board (VHPB), created, sponsored, and infiltrated by the manufacturers. In September 1998, while the dreadful hazards of the campaign had been given media coverage in France, the VHPB met a panel of "experts", the reassuring conclusion of which were extensively announced as reflecting the WHO's position: yet some of the participants in this panel had no more expertise than that of being employees of the manufacturers, and the vested interests of the rest did not receive any attention.

Even more damning: in an interview published in a widely diffused French Journal (Sciences Et Avenir, January 1997), Beecham's Business manager claimed with outrageous cynicism "we started increasing the awareness of the European experts of the WHO about hepatitis B in 1988. From the to 1991, we financed epidemiological studies on the subject to create a scientific consensus about hepatitis being a major public health problem. We were successful because in 1991, WHO published new recommendations about hepatitis B vaccination."

It is sad news for people everywhere in the world that the WHO's experts need manufacturers' salesman to become aware of significant health problems.

It should not be difficult to penetrate the morass of phony statistics, fraudulent medical hypotheses and cynical sales promotions underlying the use of hepatitis B vaccine and to focus on the individual trauma suffered by each and every casualty of such a brutally callous and useless program. Never-the-less, the hepatitis B vaccine express continues unabated--and carries us directly into the next chapter "The Death of Africa", where we enter a Kafkaesque world that none of us could have ever imagined.

CHAPTER XIX
THE DEATH OF AFRICA
The Origin of AIDS

You have arrived at what might well be called the main event in this book. Although this chapter is primarily about the death of Africa it might just as well be entitled "The Death of the World" as the AIDS epidemic spreads inexorably over the globe.

If the previous chapters have accomplished anything, I hope it has opened our minds to the truth that we shouldn't always believe in the integrity or truthfulness of government "experts". Only then do we have the basis with which to separate fact from fiction. Much of what is discussed in these remaining chapters will be described as "controversial". I submit to you that scenarios that most closely accord with the scientific facts are not controversial. What is controversial are government pronouncements which are entirely unsupported by science and totally outside of accordance with all known epidemiological facts.

The question which we will first address is relatively simple, although we will be assured that it is a matter of profound complexity involving computation of genomic mutations far beyond our capacity to understand. I assure you, however, that the answer can be resolved quite easily, well before any discussion of esoteric computer programs.

The question is; where did the AIDS virus originate? There are essentially only two possible answers. The first is that there was a natural jump (zoonosis) from an animal species to man as is proposed by the main line medical establishment. The second possibility is that AIDS is iatrogenic -- That is, it was caused by man. Did AIDS come from an African monkey or an American laboratory?

We have all heard the phrase "follow the money" in regards to penetrating nefarious agendas, but in this instance the admonition must be "follow the monkey" if we want to get to the truth. Unfortunately, a great deal of what we need to know is cloaked in secrecy and hidden in untouchable vaults. Thus, we have to rely on our own powers of observation to parse out the relevant scientific facts that fortunately are too obvious to be hidden.

As a start we must know something about the creature we are investigating - that is, the AIDS virus or HIV-1.

HIV-1 (human immunodeficiency virus) is a retrovirus and a member of the genus lentivirus. Many species are infected by lentiviruses, which are characteristically responsible for long duration illnesses with long incubation periods. Lentiviruses are RNA viruses which when they enter a host cell convert the RNA to DNA by an enzyme known as reverse transcriptase. Lentiviruses are pathogenic in a host of mammalian species including primates, sheep, goats, horses, cats, cattle, koalas, and mice. An ancestor of the lentiviruses named "RELIK" has been traced back 7 million years. Throughout all that time man has been in close contact with all of these species and butchered and eaten countless numbers of them. **Throughout the millennia of man's evolution no lentivirus has ever jumped from an animal to being pathogenic in a human being.**

Passing through these millennia of non-events brings us to 1964 and the origin of the Special Virus Cancer Program (SVCP). This research program was responsible for the development, production, seeding and deployment of various animal cancer and immuno-suppressive AIDS-like viruses and retro-viruses. These laboratory created viruses were capable of inducing disease when transferred between animal species and also when transplanted into human cells and tissue. The annual reports of the SVCP contained proof that species jumping of animal viruses was a common occurrence in labs a decade before AIDS.

Connected with the SVCP were the most famous American AIDS scientists such as Robert Gallo, Max Essex, and Peter Duesberg, (who claims HIV does not cause AIDS). Gallo and

238

Essex were also the first to promote the widely accepted African Green Monkey theory of AIDS. This theory was proven erroneous as far back as 1988, but was heavily circulated among AIDS educators and the media until the theory was superseded by the chimpanzee theory in the late 1990's.

By 1971, over 2000 primates had been inoculated at Bionetics Research Laboratories, under contract to Fort Detrick. By the early 1970's experimenters had transferred cancer causing viruses into several species of monkeys and had also isolated a monkey virus that would have a close genetic relationship to the new Kaposi's sarcoma herpes virus that would emerge in 1979 along with the AIDS virus.

Before I get too far ahead of myself, it would be useful to review testimony submitted to the House of Representatives Sub Committee on Department of Defense appropriations on Tuesday July 1, 1969; entitled; "synthetic biological agents."

"There are two things about the biological agent field I would like to mention. One is the possibility of technological surprise. Molecular biology is a field that is advancing very rapidly and many eminent biologists believe that within a period of 5 to 10 years it would be possible to produce a synthetic biological agent, an agent that does not naturally exist and for which no natural immunity could have been acquired.
MR. SIKES, are we doing any work in that field?
DR. MCCARTHUR, we are not.
MR. SIKES, why not? Lack of money or lack of interest?
DR. MCCARTHUR, certainly not lack of interest.
MR. SIKES, would you provide for our records information on what would be required and what the advantages such a program would be, the time and the cost involved?
DR. MCCARTHUR, we will be very happy to.
The following information was provided:

1. All biological agents up to the present time are representatives of naturally occurring disease and are thus known by scientists through out the world.
2. Within the next 5 to 10 years it would probably be possible to make a new infective microorganism which could differ in certain important aspects from any known disease -causing organism. Most important of these is that it might be refractory to the immunological and therapeutic processes upon which we depend to maintain our relative freedom from infectious disease.
3. A research program to explore the feasibility of this could be completed in approximately 5 years at a total cost of 10 million dollars.
4. It is a highly controversial issue and there are many who believe such research should not be undertaken lest it lead to yet another method of massive killing of large populations.

On December 15, 1969, the House Appropriations Committee passed and voted to provide the funds for the research and development of such an organism under HR 15090.

In volume 47 of the Bulletin of the WHO pages 257 -274 (1972) we find the following recommendation:

1. A systematic evaluation of the effects on viruses on immune functions should be undertaken. A number of viruses should be studies and a standard set of immune functions should be employed.
2. The effects of virus infection on different cell types (that is, macrophages, T and B lymphocytes) should be studied in greater detail with morphological changes perhaps serving as an indication of functional alterations.
3. An attempt should be made to ascertain whether viruses can in fact exert selective effects on immune function, that is, by depressing 7 S versus 19 S antibodies, or, by effecting T cell function as opposed to B cell function (Allison et. al. 1972). The possibility should also be looked into that the immune

response to the virus itself may be impaired if the infecting virus damages more or less selectively the cells responding to the viral antigen.

Thus AIDS today is the coincidental occurrence of such a virus which selectively effects T cells and is now pathogenic in humans some 7 million years after the first retrovirus was extant.

Viral recombinations (hybrids) were routinely carried out by Dr. Gallo at that time. Cross species leaps, contrary to popular belief, were not easily or spontaneously induced. To get these new man-made viruses (called "mutant hybrids") to jump species into man, the viruses were cultured in human white blood cells in some studies, and human fetal tissue cells in other studies.

It is my belief that Dr. Gallo and his team created the AIDS virus by combining the bovine leukemia virus and visna sheep virus and possibly a segment of the simian immunodeficiency virus and injecting them into human tissue cultures.

In the Journal of Theoretical Biology 2000 an article entitled "Bridging the Gap: Human diploid cell strain and the origin of AIDS" Dr. Billi Goldberg made the following observation:

"Although the theory of the chimpanzee origin of HIV-1 with cross- species transfer to man has now gained popularity, **a more likely scenario is that chimps and humans were infected by an HIV-1 precursor virus derived from a contaminated vaccine.**

The reason for the rapidity and the ease of cross-species transfer of this precursor virus has not been elucidated. We hypothesize that the vaccine was passaged in a human diploid cell strain. This simple manipulation allowed the retrovirus to adapt to human tissues and may have spawned the AIDS pandemic".

The possibility of two separate epidemics on different continents at different times-U.S. HIV-1 B strain and African HIV-1 non B strain was considered "highly unlikely" without such a bridging event having occurred.

According to comparisons done using the Los Alamos NIH Nucleotide laboratories- HIV shares 24% POL gene protein similarity to bovine leukemia virus and 33% POL gene protein similarity with bovine visna like virus.

Amazingly, in 1974, an experiment occurred in which 2 infant chimpanzees were fed milk from cows which were infected with bovine leukemia virus. These chimpanzees developed a T cell depleting leukemia and 2 years later, in 1976, they died of an immuno- deficiency disorder with symptoms of wasting, anorexia, pneumocystis carinii pneumonia, and bacterial invasion as a result of loss of T cells. The researchers highlighted that this was the first time they had ever seen P carinii associated with death in primates.

This is a documented case of intentional human - created viral immuno- deficiency disease in primates occurring nearly a decade before the recognition of HIV as the cause of AIDS. No researcher has compared this virus to HIV or has genetically sequenced the virus from the frozen sera of the chimps with AIDS.

Here is the documentation of the above experiment:

1. McClure HM, Keeling ME, - Erythroleukemia in two infant chimpanzees fed milk from cows naturally infected with the bovine C-type virus. Cancer Research 1974, October.

2. Chandler SW, McClure HM, Pulmonary Pneumocystosis in non- human primates. Arch pathol lab med. 1976 March.

Scientists are fully engaged in hunting for ancestor viruses of HIV in chimps in the African wild while totally ignoring all the immuno suppressive viruses created in virus laboratories shortly before the eruption of AIDS.

The bovine retroviruses have close similarity with the HIV virus in that they can be isolated only after cultivation in vitro and can only be transmitted congenitally, sexually, or by blood transfer.

A research article was published in Science January 11, 1985 by MA Gonda, F Wong-Staal, and RC Gallo et.al, entitled; Sequence Homology and Morphologic Similarity of HTLV-3 and Visna Virus, a pathogenic lentivirus:
    "A study was conducted of the genetic relationship between human T cell lymphotrophic retroviruses and sheep visna virus. Results obtained by molecular hybridization indicated that a greater extent of nucleotide sequence homology exists between HTLV-3 and visna virus than between HTLV-3 and any of the other viruses. The fine structure of HTLV-3 and visna virus also demonstrated striking similarities."
    Also, published in Science Magazine - March 1985 is the following article: Bovine Leukemia Virus (BLV) - related antigens in lymphocyte cultures infected with AIDS - associated viruses, L Thiry et al.:
"An earlier finding that lymphocytes from African patients with AIDS react to antigens of bovine leukemia virus prompted a study of the possible cross reactions between BLV and the AIDS virus."

Building a case for a scientific hypothesis is like building a brick wall. Each brick provides a small piece of the wall which must be laboriously constructed to reach a useful end. In science, published articles must be juxtaposed like bricks in a wall in order to attest to the work being done during the decade preceding AIDS.

It is enlightening to merely peruse a small portion of the body of publications, germane to this issue, that we can find preceding the AIDS epidemic. For a little-known disease of Icelandic sheep the visna virus was the subject of a tremendous amount of research in the 70' as well as was the bovine immunodeficiency virus. So let's scan quickly through a few of the many hundreds of studies pertaining to these viruses. The titles are informative:

1. Poly- adenylic acid in visna virus RNA 1971
2. RNA tumor virus reverse transcriptase 1973
3. DNA polymerase in human lymphoblastoid cells infected with simian sarcoma virus, BioChem Acta 1974
4. Primate type- C virus related reverse transcriptase and RNA in human leukemia cells 1974
5. Reverse transcriptase in normal rhesus monkey placenta 1974
6. Infection of human cell cultures with bovine visna virus, Georgiades JA, J Gen Vir 1978
7. Isolation of a virus from cattle with persistent lymphocytosis. Van Der Matten MJ, JNCI 1972
8. Ultra- structural studies of a visna like virus from cattle, Booth AD, J VIR 1974
9. Serological evidence of transmission of bovine leukemia virus to chimpanzees, Van Der Matten MJ, Vet Micro 1976
10. The detail structure of visna maedi virus, Harter DH, Front Biol. 1976
11. Visna virus infection of sheep and human cells in vitro, Macintyre EH, J Cell Science 1973
12. Visna-Maedi virus infection in cell cultures and in laboratory animals, Thormar H, Front Biol. 1976

13. Purification and characterization of DNA polymerase (reverse transcriptase) from two primates RNA tumor viruses, RC Gallo ,J of Virology 1973

It is clear that researchers were infecting human cells with visna virus well before AIDS broke out. Any time that you expose a virus to a new host, there is danger that the virus will adapt to that host and create a new pathogenic strain.

In January 1985, Science Magazine published an electron microscopic photograph by RC Gallo comparing HIV virus and Visna virus and showing them to be identical and indistinguishable.

A little known fact is that humans have been infected with simian immunodeficiency virus, (SIV), Bovine leukemia virus and sheep visna virus for hundreds of years without pathogenic effect. Tests for HIV infection will cross react with these viruses and will be false positive in 75% of cases unless they are diluted 400 times.

Another interesting observation is that most of the mammalian lentiviruses are spread by milk. Humans, consumers of goat's milk, sheep's milk and cow's milk have presumably been exposed to animal lentiviruses for thousands of years. It is difficult to understand how humans never became infected with a deadly disease until after the decade of massive lentivirus research.

In the decade before AIDS it was extremely common to transfer and adapt animal retroviruses and herpes viruses into human cells in genetic engineering experiments. In the process of these species-jumping experiments, scientists hybridized viruses, seeded them into various animal species, and planted them into animal and human cultures. Myriads of new laboratory-created mutant, hybrid and recombinant viruses were created, some of which were exceedingly dangerous. RC

245

Gallo, our leading virologist, has denied that such technology was possible at that time.

The danger provoked by all these laboratory-created new viruses was well known. At a symposium on leukemia research **in 1973, Danish pathologist J Clemmesen warned** that the transmissibility of **these genetically altered viral agents could cause a world epidemic** of cancer if they escaped from the laboratory.

By an almost cataclysmic conjunction of coincidences in the decade prior to the discovery of the AIDS virus, the entire repertoire of science and technology required to detect, locate, isolate and culture a retrovirus was born:
- T cells were discovered only in the 70's
- Reverse transcriptase was discovered in the 70's
- HTLV 1 and HTLV 2 retroviruses were discovered in the late 70's by RC Gallo
- A method of culturing T cells (using interleukin) was discovered in the 70's by R.C. Gallo
- The western blot and Elisa tests for detecting specific viral protein (and HIV) were discovered in the 70's

Without each and all of these discoveries it would have been impossible to discover and culture the AIDS virus HIV-1. It is extremely fortuitous that the genus lentivirus waited 7 million years to become pathogenic in man until in the 1970's when we, at last, had all the tools we needed to discover and treat the disease.

And that brings us to the first documented case of a pathogenic animal retrovirus jumping species to a human in 1978 into a San Francisco homosexual named Ken Horne. As unlikely as this trans-species jump was, it occurred simultaneously with a second unlikely trans-species jump of an entirely different virus - herpes-8; the cause of the disease of Kaposi's sarcoma. (A virus closely related to the monkey virus, herpes-Samurai).

On June 5th 1981, the CDC reported a cluster of cases of pneumocystis pneumonia in 5 gay men in Los Angeles. On July 4, 1981, the CDC again reported a cluster of Kaposi's sarcoma and pneumocystis pneumonia among gay men in San Francisco and New York City.

By the end of 1981, 121 people had died of this new disease. None of these unfortunate young men from New York, San Francisco and Los Angeles had been to Africa. None had butchered or eaten a monkey and only a handful had contact with one another. Now that AIDS has reared its ugly head exactly what were we seeing? Between 1978 and 1982 there developed approximately 9 epicenters of AIDS in the US, Haiti and Africa. These epicenters each contained 2 distinct diseases, that is, AIDS and Kaposi's sarcoma, and developed on separate continents among totally diverse populations.

The HIV strain in the US and North America is different from the predominant strains in Africa. The number of people infected within 10 years of the onset reached into the millions. Such a growth curve is epidemiologically impossible stemming from a single event or infection.

There were only 2 hypotheses as to the origin of these epidemics. The first, propounded originally by RC Gallo, is that the AIDS epidemic began when an African man contracted AIDS by eating an African green monkey. The African green monkey theory proved erroneous almost immediately, since African green monkeys harbor no viruses closely related to HIV.

It became necessary to find alternate theories, so Dr. Beatrice Hahn, an old colleague of RC Gallo from the laboratories of the 70's, announced that she had discovered the antecedent of the HIV virus in the droppings of a chimpanzee isolated in Cameroon.

247

Utilizing fragments of DNA which reacted to HIV tests in 2 frozen serum samples from the 1960's, scientists projected by computer analysis, the origin of AIDS in Africa to be around the turn of the century.

This essentially constitutes the entire scientific evidence put forward by the medical establishment to account for the aforementioned 8 epidemics of 2 diseases on multiple continents reaching millions of victims from 1978 to the present.

We will in short order see why it is vital to the mainstream medical authorities that the origin of the AIDS epidemic be predated long before its actual 1978 appearance.

In regard to the African chimpanzee hypothesis I will point out some important facts and salient studies which render this hypothesis essentially nonsensical, and made up of only junk science and wishful thinking. It hardly seems worth the trouble at this point, but I will address the African green monkey theory as proposed by Robert Gallo.--- A team of Japanese molecular biologists in 1988 concluded that there was no genetic relationship between the African green monkey virus and the AIDS virus. This was ignored for a full decade until February 1999, when the green monkey theory was debunked in a media blitz.

Scientists now point to new genetic research which point to a nearly extinct species of African chimpanzee as the origin of HIV. Many virologists pointed out that the AIDS virus doesn't appear naturally in any animal. Aside from the pronouncements of leading, government employed, virologists that AIDS in gay Americans started in Africa, the idea of a black African heterosexual disease starting in 1982 transforming itself into a white homosexual disease in the US in 1978 is a biological and epidemiological impossibility.

Following the demise of the green monkey theory government scientists put forward the chimpanzee origin

248

theory. Over time this theory changed depending on how well their claims of finding HIV positive stored blood samples held up to scrutiny. After several media blitz reports of the first AIDS patients in Africa around 1959 were discredited, the researchers settled on 2 HIV positive serums found in Kinshasa, Congo circa 1959 and 1960.

This final chapter was trumpeted by the Associated Press on October 1, 2008 in an article entitled" Origin of AIDS virus traced to 100 years ago, study finds." It reads:

"The AIDS virus has been circulating among people for about 100 years a new study suggests. Genetic analysis pushes the estimated origin of HIV back to between 1884 and 1924. Previously, scientists had estimated the origin around 1930. AIDS wasn't recognized formally until 1981 when it got the attention of public health officials in the United States. (How clever we are!)

The results appeared in Thursday's issue of the Journal Nature. Researchers note that the newly calculated dates fall during the rise of cities in Africa and they suggest that urban development may have promoted HIV's initial establishment and early spread.

Scientists say HIV descended from a chimpanzee virus that jumped to humans in Africa, probably when people butchered chimps. Many individuals were probably infected that way, but so few other people caught the virus that it failed to get a lasting foothold, researchers say.

Key to the new work was the discovery of an HIV positive sample taken from a woman in Kinshasa in 1960. It was only the second such sample to be found, the other from 1959, also from Kinshasa.

"The new work is clearly an improvement over the previous estimate of around 1930," said Dr. Anthony Fauci, Director of the National Institute of Allergy and Infectious Diseases. His institute helped pay for the work. Experts say it's no surprise that HIV circulated in humans for about 70 years before being recognized. "An infection usually takes years to produce obvious symptoms, a lag that can mask the role of the virus, and it would have infected relatively few Africans early in its spread," they said.

One can hardly suppress total astonishment at the obvious total disregard that these "experts" have for the intelligence of anyone reading this incredibly fraudulent piece of scientific information. Do they really expect everyone to believe that thousands of victims of AIDS, covered with Kaposi's sarcoma tumors, have wandered around Africa for a full century without anyone noticing-- until it came to the attention of the public health people in the United States in 1981? All of this conjecture is based on a nonsensical theory of African urbanization, a flawed computer model and two obviously false-positive old African frozen blood samples.

It should be understood that no HIV virus has ever been found in an animal or human being anywhere in the world prior to 1978 and **no animal has ever harbored an HIV virus.** The implication that an HIV positive reaction to an Elisa test is proof of the existence of an HIV virus is simply scientific fraud. HIV tests recognize protein fragments that can be from many viruses and frozen samples give notoriously high levels of false positive results.

As Dr. Rosalind Harrison wrote in New African in June 1997, "evidence that false-positives were a major problem in both stored serum samples and samples taken for population studies for HIV in Africa was available from the mid-1980's, but has been largely ignored.

Dr. A J Nahmias of Emery University published the following in the Medical Journal Lancet in May 1986: "Because of the importance of this issue we decided to test 1213 plasmas from various parts of Africa of which 818 had been obtained as far back as 1959. We have demonstrated that one individual from central Africa had been exposed to a virus similar to HIV more than a quarter of a century ago. The identity of the donor is no longer known. No evidence of the

250

infection was found in sera taken in rural areas of the Belgian Congo or South Africa (1959), Mozambique (1969), the Congo (1982)."

In the July-August 1991 Issue of the US Public Health Report, seven American doctors and researchers from the Public Health Service led by Dr. W Robert Lange concluded definitively, that frozen samples were hugely unreliable. These findings came at the end of a study tracing some American drug addicts whose blood samples, frozen since 1971 -1972 had tested positive for HIV in 1985. **All of these samples were false positives.**

The 1959 sample from Central Africa had been lying in a freezer for 39 years before the declaration that it was the mother of all AIDS. The Lexington samples that fooled the American researchers in 1985 had been frozen for only 13 years.

A study published in Human Retrovirology December 2002, by Vladamir Lukashov states the following:

"The history of the origin HIV-1 is the subject of a continuing debate; did the epidemic start in the late 70's as it was established based on the epidemiological data, or decades earlier as it has been suggested based on the analysis of nucleotide distances in the env (a viral gene sequence) gene? Our study found that the over-estimation of the age of the epidemic in the analysis of env sequences was a bias resulting from the non-clock-like evolution at nonsynonymous sites, while the estimates based on synonymous substitutions agreed with the results of epidemiological studies. "

So what Dr. Fauci of the NAIAD and his paid colleagues expect us to swallow is that thousands of AIDS cases have been wandering around Africa for a full century undetected,

251

based on 2 false positive reactions to an Elisa test and a spurious computer model. This in the face of overwhelming epidemiological evidence proving otherwise.

Beyond this---**are we to believe, and are these, so very clever, scientists of the opinion that during the entire century of European colonialism in Africa, no man from Europe had sex with one of the countless AIDS sufferers wandering around Africa unnoticed? (French, Italian, German, Portuguese, Dutch, Spanish and, of course, British).**

THE EPIDEMOLOGICAL CASE FOR AIDS AS AN IATROGENIC EVENT

Their have been no reported blood specimens anywhere in the US that were proven HIV positive prior to the epidemic in 1979. A 1989 report by Biggar found no cases of Kaposi's sarcoma in New York in young men during 1973 to 1976. But by 1985 the incidence in Manhattan had increased 850 times and in San Francisco 2000 times. The new KS virus is closely related to a monkey tumor virus that was extensively studied by researchers in the SVCP in the decade before the epidemic.

Two cardinal realities of epidemiology require that an epidemic spreads from areas of infection to areas of non-infection and that the causative organism be the same in both areas. Neither of these basic requirements is met by the "excepted theory" of HIV originating in chimpanzees in Cameroon Africa, traveling to Zaire, thence to Haiti and finally to the US. This scenario is so contrary to the facts that it doesn't even pass the laugh test.

In the EPIDEMOLOGY OF AIDS 1989 Thomas Quinn and Jonathon Mann write that the first confirmed African cases were diagnosed in European hospitals in 1983. This is 4 years after the first gay cases were diagnosed in New York City!

To prove that AIDS is not an old disease in Africa, a team of scientists led by JW Carswell tested the blood of old, sexually-inactive people living in geriatric homes in Kampala, Uganda's largest city, an epicenter of AIDS in Africa. The elderly people's blood was tested against 716 healthy, sexually-active adults living in the same city. 15% of the healthy people were positive for HIV antibodies, but none of the elderly tested positive. This 1986 study indicated HIV had not been in Uganda for a long time, as AIDS experts were proclaiming. The team concluded: the results presented here do not support the previous suggestion that the virus might have originated in Uganda; on the contrary, they indicate it arrived in the country only recently.

In 1989 another scientific team investigated HIV antibody infection among the San bush people living in Botswana. The Sans are the oldest race living in Africa. No one tested positive for HIV.

Further, compounding the supposed African origin of AIDS are reports of different strains which influence infectivity, depending on sexual preference. The American strain is subtype B which is most easily transmitted anally or by homosexual contact. If AIDS came to the US from Africa it would be a non B strain such as A or D which is transmitted vaginally or by heterosexual contact.

Probably the most obvious fact that makes it impossible that AIDS came to the US from Africa by way of Haiti as Dr. Gallo and Dr. Fauci would have us believe, is seen in the statistics of the WHO which demonstrates the following:

United States- 1981- HIV B strain -5660 cases
Haiti- 1981- HIV B strain -200 cases

253

Africa -1983- HIV non B strain -17 cases
Zaire -1983- HIV non B strain- 1 case
Cameroon- 1983 -HIV non B strain- 0 cases

It is obvious that HIV cannot have traveled backwards from the Cameroon to the US as we are being told. In fact, the first cases of AIDS were in the United States in 1978 and 1979- totaling 14. The very first cases of AIDS in Africa were diagnosed in 1982-83 and totaling 3.

As for the absurd idea that AIDS and Kaposi's patients would go unnoticed in Africa for half a century or more I refer you to the following report.
Lancet-June 1994, Aggressive Kaposi's sarcoma in Zambia, 1983. AC Bailey:
"From 1975 to 1982 between 8 and 12 new cases of Kaposi's sarcoma were seen each year in Lusaka, Zambia. The clinical presentation conformed to descriptions of endemic KS from Uganda and Kenya. 23 patients presented with Kaposi's sarcoma in 1983, **13 of these patients presented with unusual symptoms and signs.** 8 of these 13 with "atypical Kaposi's sarcoma" failed to maintain an initial response to chemotherapy and died before the end of 1983."

This publication proves beyond a doubt that the fraudulent proposition that AIDS and or Kaposi's sarcoma existed without recognition for many years in Africa is absurd. It is obvious that these patients were recognized early on, as a totally different disease entity than had ever before existed in Africa.

This brings us back to the study in the recent issue of the journal Nature in which the origin of AIDS was traced to 100 years ago. The government scientists including Dr. Worobey and other virus researchers had numerous comments about the meaning and epidemiology to be derived from this

254

study, including some closing comments by Dr. Anthony Fauci Director of NIAID.

Either these "experts" are sorely lacking in the most rudimentary understanding of epidemiological science or they are simply part of an incredibly mendacious cover up. As an example; they state that HIV descended from a chimpanzee virus that jumped to humans in Africa probably when people butchered chimps. (Which they have been doing for thousands of years) And go on to say, many individuals were probably infected that way, but so few other people caught the virus that it failed to get a lasting foothold. (Until the growth of African cities provided more chance to pass the virus to others).

This incredibly speculative scenario comes from no other than the eminent Dr. Worobey who apparently is unaware that no chimpanzee harbors an HIV virus nor can chimpanzees be infected with HIV virus. Additionally, Dr. Worobey doesn't seem to be even minimally aware that in every country and every epicenter of this epidemic the increase in numbers of those infected with HIV-1 virus followed a classical logarithmic S shaped curve with an early doubling time of 6 months which later bent to the right to a doubling time of 2 to 3 years. Therefore, it is totally impossible for his scenario, as he puts it "but so few other people caught the virus that it failed to get a lasting foothold."

The equally eminent Dr. Fauci chimes in with his comment saying it's no surprise that HIV circulated in humans for 70 years before being recognized. He also has no apparent understanding of the classic sigmoid shaped rise of HIV infection that has been observed world wide.

He also refers to the fact that the infection takes years to produce obvious symptoms, leading to a "masking" of the effect of the virus in early Africa. In making this erroneous statement he reveals that he is totally unaware that a small but significant percentage of infected persons develop AIDS within months, which makes his "masking" comment ludicrous. (not to mention the scrupulous care taken by European colonialists to avoid AIDS in Africa for 100 years!)

The only rational conclusion is not that these gentlemen are abysmally ignorant-- but that they simply are part of a cover up. Surely, our top scientists and virologists can't be so lacking in the basic epidemiological and virological knowledge that these statements portray!

Supporting of my statements about the epidemiology and rapid spread of AIDS, an extensive epidemiological survey of reported AIDS cases (WHO) was published in 2000 which strongly supports the hypothesis that the AIDS pandemic started in the USA. This survey used cumulative cases of AIDS published in the WHO epidemiology records from 1986 until January 1994.

The pattern of the African countries was compared with non-African countries using a linear-logarithmic method.

The data concludes that AIDS in Africa started in Uganda in 1982. For Congo, Kenya, Rwanda, Zaire and Zimbabwe the first year is 1983. Burundi, Central African Republic and Tanzania had the start of their national epidemic in 1984. In Botswana, Cameroon, Cote d'Iviore, Ghana, Malawi and Mozambique it started in 1986. In Ethiopia, Gabon, Nigeria and Togo it started in 1987.

The pattern shown throughout is a classic sigmoid curve and it is also noted there are always some patients that develop clinical signs almost without any latency at all.

These data put out of all question the fact that the African part of the AIDS pandemic originated in Uganda in 1982, 3 years after the origin of the world epidemic, which started in New York, USA 1978.

The first 14 AIDS patients appeared in 1979 in Manhattan. The first patients were even confined to Manhattan and Greenwich Village, and when their addresses were plotted onto a map, the New York City Blood Center was found to be the epicenter. **The Blood Center was the place where an experimental hepatitis B vaccine was tested,** using voluntary homosexual men as guinea pigs, with its start in autumn 1978.

The pattern of the epidemic was rather explosive. Within 2 years 80 patients had shown clear signs of the yet unexplained disease. In autumn of 1980 the same pattern was repeated in Los Angeles and San Francisco. For all these 3 cities there was a common dominator. Young, healthy, educated, homosexual men were enrolled in a trial testing a new hepatitis B vaccine. These trials started first in New York in November 1978 and in the California cities in March of 1980.

To verify the origin of these first viral infections the blood samples of these original patients should be obtained and genetically sequenced, however, their samples are stored in a freezer sealed by the Department of Justice.

AIDS in America clearly traces back to the US Federal Governments hepatitis B experiments performed on thousands of gay volunteers between the years 1978 to 1981 in New York City, San Francisco and Los Angeles. The vaccine was manufactured by the National Institute of Health. Also taking part in the study was the CDC in Atlanta, the NIAID and the drug companies Merck and Abbott Laboratories. 3 months after the experiment began at the NYC Blood Center the first AIDS case was discovered in a young, white Manhattan gay. To this day the NYC Blood Center refuses to release their data on the AIDS deaths. Moreover, since 1984, when 64% of the men who got the vaccine were infected with HIV, no additional reports have been released.

Despite confusing misinformation and the "puzzlement of AIDS experts" to the contrary, AIDS in Haiti began only after the hepatitis B experiments, when New York homosexual tourists took AIDS to Port Au Prince in 1979.

THE HEPATITIS B VACCINE AND AIDS IN AFRICA

Hepatitis B programs began in Africa in 1981- presaging the beginning of AIDS in Africa. The first of these programs were in Kenya, Zambia, Gambia, and Uganda. All of these countries had a first case of AIDS by 1984. Uganda was the earliest case in 1982.

In 1982 and 1983 Mozambique, Senegal, Ivory Coast, Swaziland and Zaire hosted hepatitis B vaccine program. All of these countries reported their first cases of AIDS between 1983 and 1985.

Most of the records of these programs have disappeared from the internet. However, the following examples are presented:

LANCET 1986 NOVEMBER 15 - A 7 year study of hepatitis B vaccine efficacy in infants from an endemic area (Senegal) [Due to their state authorized employment and high risk for infections; Senegalese female prostitutes were required to receive hepatitis B vaccination for relicensure. [The fact that Essex et.al. Found SIVagm, a documented vaccine contaminant, in the blood of these human subjects, is additional compelling evidence in support of the HB vaccine AIDS origination theory.]

Journal of Medical Virology 1993 - July
"9 year follow-up study of a plasma derived hepatitis B vaccine in rural African setting"
The abstract states: 101 of 255 recipients of a plasma derived hepatitis B vaccine were evaluated in 1990, 9 years after the first vaccine dose in a study in Zambia.

If one examines a map of Africa showing early AIDS incidence, one can see five rather distinct epicenters of AIDS infections with wide separation between each one.

Epicenter 1- Kenya/Uganda
Epicenter 2- Zaire/Rwanda,
Epicenter 3- Ivory Coast
Epicenter 4- Swaziland,
Epicenter 5 -Zambia/Botswana/Zimbabwe

Each of these epicenters of heavy AIDS infection was the center of a documented hepatitis B vaccine program one to two years prior. If AIDS was a naturally occurring jump of HIV and KS viruses in at least 5 separate epicenters hundreds or thousands of miles apart, the guilty chimps responsible must have been doing a hell of lot of traveling from their home base in the Cameroon!

The probability that all 8 worldwide epicenters would be the site of a hepatitis B vaccine program "coincidentally" just prior to their first AIDS cases is far less than the probability that I will be struck by lightning in the next 30 seconds, and is about equal to the probability that AIDS came from Africa to the U.S. (30 seconds have passed and I'm still conscious.)

The simplest of mathematical calculations places the probability of eight or more "starburst" epidemics of different subtypes , including two unrelated viruses, on two continents in the hundreds of millions to one--no matter how many false positive tests one does on chimp droppings in the Cameroon.

For this chapter, one major question remains: was the iatrogenic spread of AIDS accidental or deliberate? Certainly the obvious and buffoon-like cover up which followed would be in place, in either case. I will cite two relevant points concerning this question.

Why were Africans subjected to a potentially dangerous vaccine years after AIDS began in the US following its use?

Why is ALPHAMIR, a proven, effective treatment and prophylaxis for AIDS, invented by Dr. D, suppressed and ignored?

I will leave the answer to these final questions to you, the reader. Before leaving the subject of the origin of AIDS and moving on to the future of AIDS, I will leave you with this final quotation:

"It is entirely plausible that the AIDS epidemic was started in the US deliberately. Few people would need to know of the plan, and the actions of one person would be sufficient to ignite the epidemic. Maximum effectiveness would require that the introduction of an effective means of stopping the virus was blocked for as long as possible, by a carefully planned and sustained campaign of disinformation. The special problem of the release of an AIDS-like virus is that it opens up a Pandora's Box, but it is naive to believe that nobody would be willing to do so."

Dr. John Seale,
Member of the Royal College of Medicine, London,
Journal of the Royal Society of Medicine, September 1988 (volume 81 pp 537-539)

CHAPTER XX

THE DEATH OF AFRICA

Today and Tomorrow

Now that Pandora's Box has been opened and AIDS is upon us - where is it going and what can we do about it. Certainly the drug companies leave no vacuum unfilled when it comes to providing drugs and reaping profits. Providing effective and safe drugs, however, is a more elusive and sometimes unattainable goal. All the drug "breakthroughs" are accompanied by effusive hyperbole from drug companies and media alike. This scenario was never more the case than with the explosive debut of AZT (zidovudine) to all those desperately waiting for an AIDS cure. No one doubted that modern science would triumph, and that the answer to AIDS was at hand. The only thing not forthcoming was a parade of marching bands.

The story of AZT is more than enlightening. It is a sad microcosm of the gigantic façade of the supercilious aristocracy of medicine claiming the high ground of moral and scientific superiority -- only to find themselves standing knee deep in mud.

It was little known at that time that AZT was a metabolic poison purposely designed by Dr. Richard Beltz in 1961 to kill blood cells for the use as cancer chemotherapy.

Since the introduction of AZT as an AIDS drug in 1987, following a grossly corrupt clinical trial, hundreds of research papers have reported AZT to be profoundly toxic to all cells of the human body. The original phase 1 trial that was conducted to see whether humans could endure the drug's toxicity, showed a short term death rate of 33%. The conclusion was made that AZT was safe enough, and Glaxo Smith Kline immediately went forward with the pivotal phase 2 AZT licensing trial.

At the point that the phase 2 trial was terminated (4 months), 19 out of the 137 member placebo group had died, against only 1 of the 145 patients administered AZT. On this basis the FDA licensed AZT for the treatment of AIDS.

Despite these impressive findings a critical look at the study showed marked corruption and irregularity. To begin

262

with, many of the patients were on the protocol for only a few weeks. FDA inspectors reported irregularities that biased against the placebo group. The trial rapidly became unblinded; neither doctors nor patients were supposed to know who was on treatment and who was on placebo. The study was prematurely terminated after 17 weeks, as the study was unblinded, and doctors knew that more people were dying in the placebo group than the treated group.

The strange thing about this trial was that patients in the control group officially on sugar pill placebos, also suffered from AZT's toxic effects. Many of the placebo patients along with the AZT treated group needed repeated blood transfusion to survive. **It was obvious that the patients were sharing the real drug.**

TAC (Treatment Action Campaign) Executive President Zackie Achmat, TAC Chairman and AIDS Law Project Director Mark Heywood, and Judge Edwin Cameron - flayed the multi- center clinical trials of AZT as the sloppiest, most poorly controlled trial ever to serve as the basis for an FDA Licensing approval.

In no other clinical trial were the fabulous results of this phase II study ever reproduced. As a matter of fact, all major subsequent studies demonstrated that those who took AZT got sicker and died quicker than those who didn't.

In 1990, the AIDS clinical trial group that did the original phase II study undertook and published a second study known as the half dose trial. This study was published in the NEJM (New England Journal of Medicine) in October 1990.

The extreme toxicity which AZT users were suffering from, including massive anemia requiring multiple blood transfusion and a horrendous death rate, impelled Dr. Fischel and the her AIDS clinical trial group to do a study comparing the full dose of AZT with a half dose of AZT, hoping it would show a reduction in toxicity -- the sad fact was that all the

263

original test subjects from the phase II trial (the placebo group were put on AZT as well) were dead by the end of 1989.

So let's take a close look at the infamous half dose study of October 1990. (A study which I present to you as one of the most egregious insults to the intelligence of the medical community in the history of science, never-the-less, they bought it.)

A RANDOMIZED CONTROL TRIAL OF A REDUCED DAILY DOSE OF AZT: OCTOBER 11, 1990 NEJM
We will first look at what the authors had to say about this study in the preliminary abstract:

"The initially tested dose of AZT for treatment of patients with AIDS was 1500 mg. **Although this dose is effective, it is associated with substantial toxicity.**

Results: the median length of follow up was 25 months. At 18 months the estimated survival rates were 52% for the standard treatment group and 63% for the low dose group. At 24 months the estimated survival rate was 27% for the standard group and 34% for the low dose group. In both groups, 82% of the subjects had another opportunistic infection.

Conclusion: the reduced daily dose of AZT was at least as effective as the standard dose and was less toxic."

The most obvious and amazing outcome of this study was that both groups were on AZT, and the death rate in both groups exceeded the death rate of the placebo group in the original phase II trial that purported to show a higher death rate in the placebo group than in the treatment group. In other words, at this point these **researchers knew beyond doubt, that AZT was not only not working but was killing people faster than no treatment at all.**

264

More-over, of the 524 subjects enrolled (all on AZT treatment) only 41 completed the study. All the rest developed a major opportunistic infection, tumor, intolerable toxic reaction or death. The survival rate in both groups was less than 5% at 32 months.

I submit to you that no objective evaluation of these atrocious results should lead a researcher or physician to continue recommending the use of AZT for the treatment of AIDS. It is unconscionable that the abstract states that 1500 mg. of AZT is an effective treatment for AIDS. Even though, it was clear from these data that the initial study was totally wrong.

The final study which should have ended the AZT myth was the Anglo-French CONCORDE trial published in Lancet 1994. The CONCORDE study went on for 3 years examining 1749 HIV positive people against a placebo control. The team concluded that: "AZT is a highly toxic and carcinogenic drug, which neither prolongs life nor staves off symptoms of AIDS, in people who are HIV positive but have not yet progressed to AIDS." **The study clearly demonstrated a significantly increased risk of death of people on AZT compared with placebo.**

If CONCORDE appeared surprising, it was because those in the US had been captivated by a self- induced AZT mythology. Dr. Anthony Fauci, Director of the NIAID recommended that any one with HIV antibodies and less than 500 CD-4 cells should start taking AZT at once. At that time, that meant 650 thousand people in the US.

The CONCORDE team was put under tremendous pressure from Burroughs Welcome and US researchers to terminate the trial, as they claimed that it was" unethical" to conduct a trial using a placebo group, since AZT had already been "proven" effective. When asked about this, Dr. Ian

265

Weller, a chief investigator of CONCORD stated, "yes, there has been pressure, and it has been placed at the very highest levels."

Despite the failure of AZT in these trials [and many others], AZT mono -therapy remained in place, with hardly a murmur of dissent until the advent of triple therapy and HAART (highly active anti- retroviral therapy) beginning in 1996. Just what we would expect from a totally compliant medical establishment.

Before we launch into the modern era of AIDS drugs - that is the nucleoside and non- nucleoside cocktails as well as the protease inhibitors - I must reiterate the fact that no amount of statistical and clever manipulation of clinical trials or media hype can substitute for a properly done, placebo controlled clinical trial. Drug companies and researchers call it "unethical" to do a placebo controlled trial when a "proven" treatment exists. What is really unethical is to allow them to use this excuse to foist useless and dangerous drugs upon us, ad infinitum. The result is literally hundreds of drugs being rushed into the market without any real proof of their efficacy or safety.

This is exactly where we stand today in regard to the ever growing pipeline of anti-AIDS drugs. These drugs have an absolute consensus of validity. No one questions and their lifesaving virtues are trumpeted daily by an adoring media and all medical "experts". The well understood toxicity limitations of chemotherapy agents so long accepted in cancer therapy are out the window. Chemotherapy is now an acceptable lifelong "maintenance" program. Side effects be damned.

Does this sound familiar? Exactly what we heard for a full decade about the wonder drug AZT. One might be allowed to ask the question, how it is possible that three drugs which are individually ineffective can become, suddenly, massively effective when combined into a "cocktail"? Despite the overwhelming consensus of the scientific community, (a condition which I have long ago learned is of no scientific validity what- so- ever,) I consider it more than useful to look into the possibility that, as we have seen so many times before, these drugs do not work as well as being touted and perhaps do not work at all.

The primary purported proof of the efficacy of HAART is the post 1995 precipitous drop in the AIDS death rate attributed to the drugs which were approved and became available in 1995. The first serious problem with this contention is that the death rate began its precipitous drop long before these drugs were in wide-spread use.

The decline in death from 1995 to 1996 was 25% while less than 1% of AIDS patients had a prescription for these new drugs.

From 1996 to 1997 the death rate declined an additional 42% while less than 17% of AIDS patients in the US were on the new drugs.

From 1997 to 1998 there was an additional 33% decrease in the death rate. In that year, the number of patients on the new drug rose to 40% (Lancet 2003, October 18th.)

From 1998 thru 2002 when an additional 40% of AIDS patients went on the cocktail there was no further decrease in AIDS deaths!

It is hard to understand how such a major decrease in death rate could be due to these drugs if 67% of the drop occurred prior to their distribution. It is also difficult to understand why the additional use of these drugs from 40% to nearly 80% had no effect what-so- ever on the death rate!

267

Despite this troublesome statistical reality, these drugs were universally credited with being the cause of the reduction in death rate. Dr. Helene Gayle of the CDC noted that "in a period of 2 years, new combination treatments cut the annual level of deaths in half, but it appears that most of the benefit of the new treatments has been realized." She obviously failed or was unwilling to recognize that the majority of the drop occurred before these drugs were in use and, more astonishingly, she doesn't have an explanation for why there was no additional drop in the death rate when an additional 50% or more of patients went on these drugs.

Of course, since she was unaware of these facts, it must have never occurred to her that the drop in the death rate seen in men was not in any-way matched by the decline in death rate in women. No-where have I seen any one question how a drug cocktail could be so effective in men and not work in women. The fact is, that there was only a concomitant slight drop in the death rate of women starting in 1995 and leveling off in 1997. Since 1997, **despite massive increase in cocktails there has been no drop whatsoever in the death rate male or female!**

In the journal American Medical Association 2008, it was stated that only 17% of AIDS patients were started on the new therapy between 1996 and 1997 when the AIDS death rate had already fallen nearly 90%.

Are we again looking at assumptions and speculations by the AIDS experts that are not backed by real data? We are again faced with the problem of failure of the scientific establishment to do the proper placebo controlled trials necessary to separate fact from hype and media blitz.

Looking further, at data which may give us indications of the real effectiveness of these drugs, we find a University of California published article entitled "AIDS cocktail therapy helps even the most advanced patients ":

268

Despite this positive sounding title, in this study the death rate of advanced AIDS patients on HAART was 23% per year. This death rate is worse than it was in 1990 on AZT mono-therapy!

To give us a basis upon which to evaluate the true effect of HAART, let's first look at a cohort of AIDS patients that were followed over a ten year period in the pre- HAART era. These data were presented at the International AIDS Conference in 1994.

The cumulative mortality at 11.5 years was 46% or 4% per year. The highest death rate was in the 10th year at 7%. There were 0 deaths in the first 2 years (it should be noted that persons starting on HAART today do so within less than 2 years of sero- conversion).

Data from a cohort of HIV positive persons on HAART in China show a continuous death rate of 5% per year over a 6 year period.

Published in Chemotherapy 2000 by Funk, et al: "Mortality rate with advanced HIV/AIDS using new ARV therapies". In this study there were 160 deaths over 1225 person- years for an annual death rate of 13%.

In a joint study from Baltimore and Rio de Janeiro 2545 HIV/AIDS patients were followed for 2 years. The death rate in this cohort was 4.5% per year.

Of course, the death rate in any particular cohort or group will be very closely associated with the severity of their illness at the time of observation. It is therefore difficult to compare pre and post HAART cohorts; however, there seems to be, on the data presented, little difference to be noted between the death rates today and the 4% seen in the study prior to 1995. Moreover, if we examine the real world death rates on

HAART treatment in Africa we find little reason to believe that these drugs are as effective as everyone is trying to make us believe.

THE ANTIRETROVIRAL THERAPY COHORT COLLABORATIVE, - LANCET 2006

"The results of this collaborative study which involved 20 thousand patients with HIV-1 from Europe and North America show that the virological response (viral load) after starting HAART has improved steadily since 1996. **However, there was no corresponding decrease in the rate of AIDS, or deaths up to 1 year of follow up.** Conversely, there was some evidence for an increase in the rate of AIDS. We noted a discrepancy between the clear improvement we recorded for virological response and the apparent worsening rate of clinical progression."

LANCET EDITORAL COMMENTS:
"The major findings are that, despite improved initial HIV virological control there were no significant improvements in early immunological response as measured by CD4 lymphocyte count, no reduction in all cause mortality, and a significant increase in combined HIV/AIDS- related death risk."

And in Africa:

INFORMATION FOR DEPARTMENT OF HEALTH MEDIA LIAISON OFFICER MAUPI MONYEMANGENE, 6 OCTOBER 2005

"These data revealed a perfect linear relationship between the death rate of people taking ARV's and the duration of their treatment; and they predict that within 7 years everyone on ARV's will be dead. The high treatment dropout rate reflected by these data is consistent with numerous published reports on the unendurable toxicity of ARV's for most people."

UN CONCERNED ABOUT MALAWI'S RISING DEATHS OF AIDS PATIENTS ON ARV'S, CHINA PEOPLES DAILY ONLINE, 1 NOVEMBER 2006

"United Nations special envoy for HIV/AIDS in Africa Stephen Lewis expressed concern on Tuesday over Malawi's rising number of deaths among people receiving HIV/AIDS treatment in the country. Lewis was speaking at the end of his 3 day visit to the Southern African country when he was briefed by Malawian government officials that the country was grappling with an 11% death rate of people who are receiving free anti- retroviral drugs."

SOUTH AFRICA-GOVERNMENT AIDS PROGRAM

"The western cape report shows that: out of total of 4251 patients enrolled in 3 months a total of 207 (4.8%) patients died. Out of the total of 2715 patients enrolled in 6 months, a total 196 (7.2%) patients died. Out of the 914 patients enrolled in 12 months a total of 114 (12.4%) patients died.

PATIENT RETENTION IN ANTIRETOVIRAL THERAPY PROGRAM IN SUB-SAHARIAN AFRICA: A SYSTEMATIC REVIEW. ROSEN S. ET AL. PLOS MED. OCTOBER 2007

"We conducted a systematic search of the English language published literature and conference abstracts between 2000 and 2007. We included 32 publications reporting on 33 patient cohorts totaling 74,289 patients in 13 countries in our analysis. Under the worst case scenario, 76% of patients would be lost by 2 years. The mid point scenario predicted patient retention of 50% by 2 years. The attrition comprised mainly deaths and losses to follow up. A recent attempt to trace patients in Malawi determined that 50% had died, 27% could not be found and the rest had stopped ARV's."

An excellent (in my opinion) article by Rodney Richards entitled,

NEW STUDY SHOWS AIDS DRUGS EQUALLY EFFECTIVE AS POVERTY AND MALNUTRITION:

"If antiretroviral drugs are dramatically improving survival in those infected with HIV, then shouldn't we see dramatically reduced survival in those who have no access to these drugs?

Surprisingly, this is not what is observed. In the March 8, 2002 issue of the journal AIDS, scientists from the Medical Research Council, and the Uganda virus Research Institute in Uganda (MRC/UVRI), report that untreated Ugandans are surviving "considerably longer than has been expected."
    In fact, this is an understatement. **The untreated Ugandans in the above study are actually surviving just as long as their medicated counterparts in the developed world, according to data published in the April 1, 2000 issue of The Lancet.** This latter study was conducted by the Collaborative Group on AIDS Incubation and HIV Survival Group (Collaborative Group), which analyzed data from 13,030 individuals (with known dates of seroconversion) from Europe, North America, and Australia to estimate time from seroconversion to AIDS and death.
    Specifically, **"median time from seroconversion to death was 9.8 years" in the Ugandan study, as compared to 10.1 years for aged matched individuals in the Collaborative Group study; and** median time from seroconversion to AIDS was 9.4 and 9.3 years for the two studies, respectively.
    Even more miraculously, for individuals infected at age 15-24 in these studies, 10-year survival was substantially better in antiretroviral-free Ugandans than it

272

was in their medicated counterparts living in Europe, North America and Australia (78 vs. 66%).

Could it be that these particular rural Ugandans are living in abundance with good nutrition and the necessary resources to provide for an environment conducive to fending off the opportunistic infections waiting to take advantage of their failing immune systems?

The authors give us the answer in a separate report, which was published two months earlier under the covers of a different journal (BMJ). "Most of the population: in their study area "lives in poverty; food is often in limited supply, there is no electricity, and there is poor access to any, let alone clean, water. Malaria is endemic, and infections other than HIV, especially bacterial infections, are common."

Interestingly, the BMJ publication doesn't even talk about time to AIDS or death. Rather it focuses on symptoms in these HIV infected individuals and paradoxically concludes," disease progression associated with infection with HIV-1 seems to be rapid in rural Uganda." Only in the world of HIV/AIDS can "rapid" disease progression be correlated with "considerably longer" survival. The apparently schizophrenic conclusions in these two publications, which are derived from the same patient population.

The authors of the Ugandan study attempt to divert attention from the extraordinary survival rates observed in their subjects by emphasizing they are, "comparable to survival times in industrialized countries *prior* to the widespread use of antiretroviral therapy." (*emphasis* mine) Well, this is technically true, but only because survival times haven't changed since the widespread use of antiretroviral therapy!

The Collaborative Group study analyzed data for 13,030 individuals who seroconverted in the pre-HIV-era (before 1983), the prophylaxis-era (1983-1987), the AZT-era (1987-1990), the monotherapy-era (1990-1993, and the combination therapy-era (1993-1996); and contrary to all expectations, they

273

inform us, [we]found no evidence of a difference in survival or time to the diagnoses of AIDS for individuals who seroconverted in 1983-96."

How can this be? First, we were told prophylaxis against PCP and MAC slows progression to AIDS and death, then we were told AZT dramatically slows progression to AIDS and death further yet, and then we were told combination therapy dramatically slow progression to AIDS and death even further yet! But, what do we see when we put all of this additive benefit together? Absolutely nothing!

Well, this is not quite true, for there was one group in the Collaborative Group study that did enjoy significantly better survival; namely, those who seroconverted before 1983. So technically, it is not fair to say prophylaxis, mono-therapy, and combination therapy did "nothing." Those who seroconverted in years when these drugs were immediately available actually did significantly worse. The authors offer the following incoherent rationalization to account for this: "the apparently better survival for individuals seroconverting before 1983 may be an artifact, because these individuals seroconverted before the discovery of HIV-1 as the causative agent for AIDS."

Rather than focusing on the fact that their data offers 13,030 examples demonstrating a complete lack of benefit to any of the antiretrovirals used alone or in combination up to 1996, the authors instead present this data as a summary of the situation, "before the widespread use of [HAART]." Apparently holding out the implication that now things are most certainly different. Yet the authors offer no data of their own, or even a reference to a single publication, which tells us how patients who seroconverted In the HAART era are doing.

Today, nearly two years later, the PubMed data base still lists no published comments on the results of the Collaborative Group study; and I am still unaware of any publication that reports data for survival or time to AIDS in persons with known dates of seroconversion after 1996, in the era of ostensibly better HAART therapy.

274

Even if such data were to become available, and even if the data looked good, we are still left with the fact that the 513,486 AIDS patients reported to the CDC prior to 1996, needlessly consumed billions of dollars worth of useless antiretrovirals that seriously compromised their quality, and perhaps even quantity, of life.

Do these more than half-million individuals, or their families and loved ones, deserve to know that all the promised benefits of these drugs, which were aggressively promoted by the pharmaceutical industry, our public health institutions, and uncritical journalists, were nothing more than illusions? That the only thing real that resulted from their dedicated compliance to consuming these chemicals was the compromised quality of life and debilitating side-effects they suffered? Or do we simply marginalize and divert attention from their senseless pain and suffering by shining the light of hope on the new unproven drugs of the HAART-era?

Aside from the tragic story implicit in the results of the Collaborative Group study; they do, never the less, help us understand why untreated Ugandans are surviving just as long as their infected counterparts in the developed world. Namely, according to the Collaborative group study, the drugs are demonstrably worthless at best. But still, even if these drugs are worthless, shouldn't HIV positive Americans and Europeans who have full access to food, water and health care still be doing far better than their impoverished Ugandan counterparts? Is there anything that can explain the remaining part of this paradox?

The Ugandans enrolled in the above studies did have access to regular check-ups, diagnostic testing, and free medication for routine health-care, which might have contributed to survival. However, when the researchers studied matched HIV positives outside of the study cohort, who did not have access to these amenities, survival times were no different. A "disappointing" finding for which, "we do not have a good explanation" according to the authors.

275

Perhaps access to health-care and medicine is of little use to the malnourished with no access to food or clean water?

Perhaps it might be possible that the Ugandans in these studies are not surviving surprisingly long, but rather, the subjects in developed countries on antiretroviral are actually dying surprisingly fast. Perhaps these antiretrovirals are not worthless, but are actually harmful to the same degree as poverty and malnutrition.

To check this hypothesis, I would propose giving some of the Ugandans in the above studies access to food and water. I would predict we would see their median survival significantly surpass that of their medicated counterparts in the developed world. It's not unethical to give Africans food is it? Summary:

Median time from seroconversion to AIDS and death in poor, starving rural Africans (without access to health care, purified water, electricity or drugs) living in the Masaka District of Uganda (where malaria, dysentery and measles are endemic) is no different than that observed in Europeans, North Americans, or Australians who have full access to proper nutrition, health-care, "live-prolonging" antiretrovirals, and prophylaxis against opportunistic infection."

It seems that we have at last found the placebo control group we have been pleading for--in impoverished Uganda-- and the European and North American ARV treatment cohort didn't fare well against them!

To bring us up to date on this issue we see a study published in February 2009, with the usual misleading title,

STARTING HAART EARLIER MIGHT REDUCE MORTALITY RATES, STUDY SAYS: this in the Kaiser Daily HIV/AIDS report.

276

Brinkhoff and colleagues collected data on 2-year mortality rates among HIV positive people taking HAART in Cote d'Ivoire, Malawi, South Africa and Zimbabwe. There were 1177 deaths over 14,695 person-years of follow-up. **The death rate was 8% per year.**

Those with advanced HIV had a mortality rate 500 times greater than the general population over the first three months of treatment. Even those with T4 cell counts of over two hundred, had a mortality rate 30 times higher than the general population during the first 3 months! (So much for the optimistic title!)

Looking back at our previously cited study of AIDS mortality rates by Kraib KJ et al presented at the International AIDS Conference (from the UBC AIDS Centre in Vancouver, Canada,) we can compare the death rates. This presentation was in 1994, prior to the availability of ARV's or HAART.

In that cohort over 11 years, the cumulative death rate was 4% per year. The single highest death rate of 7% was in year 10. Therefore the death rate according to this study, prior to HAART,
was half the death rate of 8% reported in the Kaiser report of February 2009.

Unfortunately, we have not yet found proof of the effectiveness of HAART, so let's look elsewhere to see if we can find statistical support. If ARV's are indeed prolonging lives then certainly the median age of AIDS deaths must increase. According to general agreement, antiretroviral treatment has yielded substantial extension of life to people diagnosed with AIDS.

As with so many other contentions of orthodox HIV/AIDS belief, however, this expectation is contrary to actual facts. The greatest risk of death from HIV disease comes at ages in the range of 35-45, just as at the beginning of the AIDS era. There was no dramatic increase in the median age of death after 1996 following the adoption of HAART.

From annual "health", United States reports: CDC: AGE DISTRIBUTION OF AIDS DIAGNOSES AND DEATHS, 1982-2004
Mean age of death 1996 39 years
Mean age of death 1998 41 years
Mean age of death 2000 42 years
Mean age of death 2001 43 years

The slow and steady increase in median age of AIDS deaths shows no pronounced upward turn following 1996- even though the annual number of deaths decreased by more than half between 1994 and 1998. The slope of the curve is essentially unchanged from 1980 onward suggesting that this slow increase after 1996 is related to factors other than the use of ARV's.

Since we can get no corroboration of the success of ARV's from age of death statistics, lets look at the overall death statistics published yearly by UNAIDS. UN AIDS estimates the number of HIV cases world wide at 33 million. This was recently revised downward from a figure of 40 million, largely due to revised methodology of estimation in India. For our purposes let's assume the figure of 40 million is correct.

The proportion of HIV positives that have reached the state of AIDS is approximately 25% of the total, or 10 million persons.

Almost all of the 2 million annual AIDS deaths are in this latter group, indicating a 20% AIDS death rate per year for AIDS globally.

Since there are now 4 million AIDS people on ARV's with a purported 80% reduction in death rate, this should translate into an 80% reduction in the 20% death rate of those

4 million -or a new death rate of 4%. A difference of 16% X 4 million or 640,000 lives saved each year!

The actual number of decreased deaths was one hundred thousand, from all causes, for the year. There was hardly a sufficient impact on the total, to warrant the glowing testimonials given to the new era of AIDS drugs. So this approach doesn't work either.

The slow decline of AIDS-related deaths is "dismally disappointing," said Selina Lo, Medical Coordinator for Doctors without borders. She said the numbers are evidence that strategies need to change.

If these new drugs are not responsible, what factors could have led to this major decline in the AIDS death rate?

Rather than correlating with the introduction of HAART, increased survival rate among AIDS patients correlate with many other factors including: improved treatment for individual opportunistic infections, declining doses of toxic drugs like AZT, DDI and 3TC, as well as, a marked decline, years earlier, in new AIDS infections, which made the later decline in death rates highly predictable.

Another primary reason for the observed increased survival in AIDS patients can be found in the ever-changing definition of what AIDS is. By definition, prior to 1993 100% of AIDS patients had one or more life threatening diseases. After January 1993, a patient was classified as an AIDS case even without any symptoms or diseases when his T4 cell level went below 200. As a result of the redefinition, in 1997, 60% of the reported AIDS cases were free of any life threatening disease.

Obviously if we were to compare survival rates between 2 groups, one where 100% of patients are deathly ill, and the other were only 39% are deathly ill, overall survival will be better in the latter group, or stated more precisely , survival should be 2.5 times better in the latter group.

Recognizing these facts, a group of researchers from the Instituto Superiore De Sanita in Rome, applied either the 1987 CDC definition, or the 1993 CDC definition to the same patient population (3515 patients from 1987 to 1991) to see what effect the definition would have on median survival times.

They discovered, "while the median survival of patients meeting the 1987 definition was 24 months, at the end of 57 months 53% of patients meeting the 1993 definition were still alive." (Vella S, et al JAMA 1994) **In other words, by simply applying the 1993 definition to the same group of patients, median survival time went up 2.5 fold.**

It is also interesting to note that median survival time in this study (using the 1993 definition) is approximately 60 months, while the median survival time reported in a New York Times article (after the benefits of new AIDS drug) is only 46 months. In other words, median survival time has dropped by over a year since the introduction of protease inhibitors in 1996.

The CDC stopped publishing how many new AIDS cases were due to non- illness at the end of 1997. As such, we will no longer know what percentage of AIDS is due to actual illness and therefore, can no longer estimate how much survival time should increase, simply due to the increased percentage of non-illness.

Since those with illness die off much faster than those without illness, the AIDS pool will continue to be enriched with non- ill patients and the survival times should continue their upward trend.

Despite all of this obvious statistical manipulation, the true story is demonstrable in the continuing reports of excessive mortality of patients initiating antiretroviral therapy.

EXCESSIVE EARLY MORTALITY IN THE FIRST YEAR OF TREATMENT IN HIV INFECTED PATIENTS INITIATING ANTIRETROVIRAL THERAPY IN

RESOURCE - LIMITED SETTINGS - UCSS Institute For Global Health, August 2008 Marizzi MC, et al.

Subjects were 3456 patients from January 2003 to December 2005 with at least 180 days of follow up since HAART initiation. In the first year of HAART, 260 deaths were recorded - 97 per 1000 person/years or 9.7%. When the mortality rate was stratified according to CD 4 cell values it was 10% in subjects with less than 200 cells, 5% in subjects with more than 200 cells, 4.4% in subjects with more than 350 cells and 2.8% in subjects with more than 500 cells. (These death rates are considerably higher than claimed to be observed among patients in high - income countries. An almost 3% death rate in persons with normal T cell levels is unheard of even prior to HAART).

Two areas that are to a large extent ignored amid the optimistic euphoria surrounding each new drug "breakthrough", are toxicity and the emergence of resistant strains. The toxicity problem is ignored because in all probability, if people knew the true risk/benefit ratio of these drugs they probably would simply refuse to take them.

The second problem is drug resistance, which is in the long run, the single most important factor to be considered. It is a mathematical certainty that HIV mutates at an incredibly fast rate-perhaps as much as a million times faster than any other virus. This makes the failure of the entire ARV program a mathematical certainty. No matter how many people are treated; no matter how much money is spent the final effect will be the terminal extermination of black Africa and, perhaps, the rest of the world as well.

When the first line drugs fail (failure means resurgence of viral load), which happens almost half the time, the problem of drug "resistance" is invoked as the culprit. This accomplishes 2 things - it removes the onus of "ineffective" and, better yet, it allows the implementation of second line or salvage therapy, using different and much more expensive drugs. No one seems to notice or mind that second line or even third line courses of therapy have a death rate considerably worse than no therapy at all!

COMPARISON OF FIRST LINE ANTIRETROVIRAL THERAPY WITH SECOND LINE REGIMEN INCLUDING NEVIRAPINE, EFAVIRENZ, OR BOTH DRUGS, PLUS STAVUDINE AND LAMIVUDINE.

"Treatment failure occurred in 96 (43.6%) of 222 patients assigned nevirapine once daily, 169 (43.7%) of 387 assigned nevirapine twice daily, 151 (37.8%) of 400 assigned efavirenz, and 111 (53.1%) of 209 assigned nevirapine plus efavirenz."

DUAL CLASS DRUG REISTANCE PRESENT IN 2/3 OF SOUTH AFRICAN HIV COHORT ON FAILING ART - CLINICAL INFECTIOUS DISEASES MAY 2008

"Almost 2/3 of individuals failing first line ART in a KawaZulu - Natal cohort had resistance to drugs from 2 classes, and 1/3 had at least one mutation that could reduce response to the entire nucleoside analog class." Second line treatment in these resistant individuals can cost 10 times as much as first line treatment. Virus samples from 83.5% of participants carried one or more significant drug resistance mutations. Dual-class drug resistance virus was present in 64.3% of participants.

GOETZ MB ET AL. EFFECT OF HIGHLY ACTIVE ANTIRETROVIRAL THERAPY ON OUTCOMES IN VETERANS MEDICAL CENTERS - AIDS MARCH 2001

"Of some concern, however, is the observation that despite increased pharmaceutical usage, the total mortality has not decreased since the first quarter of 1997. The virological failure of up to 60% of treatment-experienced patients and the increased recognition of the toxicity of antiretroviral therapy suggests that substantial additional

282

medical cost will eventually accrue in the care of these patients."

IN US CITIES, SUCCESSFUL HIV TREATMENT RARE. REUTERS. FEBRUARY 7, 2001

"One of the first studies to look at the success of HIV treatment in inner-city patients from the time of diagnoses reveals a dire situation, a doctor working in Atlanta, Georgia said here on Tuesday at the 8th Conference on Retroviruses. His study found that only one in 10 patients newly diagnosed with HIV achieved a reduction in virus in blood to "undetectable" levels - a major goal of treatment. One year after being diagnosed, 24 patients (18%) had died. One year from diagnosis only 23 were still on therapy and 12 (of the original 135 patients) had undetectable levels of virus in their blood."

AIDS. 2008 OCTOBER 1ST. LAWN SD ET AL: EARLY MORTALITY AMONG ADULTS ACCESSING ARV'S IN SUB-SAHARAN AFRICA

"Immunological and virological responses to ART are similar to responses in patients treated in high - income countries. Despite this, however, early mortality rates in sub-Saharan African are very high; **between 8 and 26% of patients die in the first year of ARV treatment, with most deaths occurring in the first few months."**

Although causes of death traditionally associated with HIV/AIDS continue play a dominant role, other conditions, including diabetes, cardiovascular disease, cancer, liver and renal diseases have been increasingly reported. The average yearly increase of non HIV associated causes of death in the HIV group was 8%. **In an HIV outpatient study, Palella et al. showed that non - HIV/AIDS related causes of death increased from 13.1% to 42.5% between 1996 and 2004 in 12 clinics in the United States,** with cardio-vascular disease being the leading cause of death in this group. (It would appear that the toxicity chickens are now coming home to roost in the ARV treated population).

Cancer rate are also increasing in this population. Colon cancer is 18 times normal, Hodgkin's disease 18 times normal, liver cancer 5 times normal, testicular cancer, melanoma, oral pharyngeal cancer and lung cancer all 2 to 3 times the normal.

While we are at it, lets take a quick look at the greater than 100% toxicity rate of ARV therapy which includes; anemia, neutropenia, liver failure, pancreatitis, lipodystrophy, thrombocytopenia, neuropathy, osteomalacia, anorexia, nausea and vomiting.

AIDS patients on HAART have a greater than 100% rate of toxicity. A commonly used drug Combivir (lamivudine + zidviudine) caused 18 adverse reactions having an incidence of between 7 and 30% each.

The overwhelming message from the data available on the new era drug cocktails is that there is sufficient evidence to cast doubt on the overwhelming consensus of efficacy that they have enjoyed. If it turns out that they are truly effective and safe despite this - it would be a clear and anomalous departure from the almost total failure of many other highly touted drugs and vaccines - and consequently, a total surprise.

Until these drugs are submitted to a proper, placebo controlled, clinical trial with matched cohorts, the final answer will remain obscured. Until a Concorde-like study is done, as it was for AZT - no one will have the necessary standing to champion the use of these drugs.

And now - a very short look at the future of AIDS.

In the decades ahead, the center of the global HIV/AIDS pandemic is set to shift from Africa to Eurasia. The death toll in that region's 3 pivotal countries - Russia, India, and China - could be staggering. This will assuredly be a humanitarian tragedy, but it will be much more than that.

The disease will alter the economic potential of the region's major states and the global balance of power.

A news item from the "The Guardian" had this to say on 7/6/2004:

"The lethal spread of the HIV/Aids pandemic across the globe is speeding up, in spite of intensifying efforts on the part of UN agencies, the US, Britain and other European governments to turn the tide. A record five million people were infected by the virus last year and nearly three million died. The UN's latest bi-annual report on the state of the pandemic made it plain yesterday that the HIV virus that causes AIDS is defeating man's best efforts to contain it. There are 38 million people carrying the virus, sub-Saharan Africa is being devastated, and the fastest spread is in Asia and Eastern Europe. "More people than any previous year became infected with HIV. That is clearly a failure to reach the people who need it with prevention methods. More people than ever before died of AIDS. That is a failure to reach them with treatment," said Peter Piot, executive director of UNAIDS, at the launch of the report in London yesterday. The epidemic, he said, is reaching its global phase, and is no longer a problem largely confined to sub-Saharan Africa. One in every four new infections is occurring in Asia, where huge populations are at risk, said the report, and published just before the international AIDS conference in Bangkok. There has been a sharp increase in the numbers infected in China, Indonesia and Vietnam, while India alone has 5.1 million people with HIV - the second largest number infected in any country, after South Africa."

In an attempt to impact the dire future of this holocaust I have contacted innumerable persons who are in a position to help initiate new strategies. This includes highly placed political figures, AIDS activists, researchers and celebrities of great stature, world wide. The following letter is an example:

September 2, 1008

285

His Excellency Ambassador Gordon Wavamuno, Uganda

Dear Ambassador Wavamuno,

I am a physician who has participated in the development of a new technology utilizing a one, two, four - Trioxolane as an antiviral, antimicrobial, and immunostimulatory agent (ALPHAMIR). I have been working as Chief Director of Research at the Kenya Medical Research Institute to complete clinical trials for both AIDS and Arthritis.
We received regulatory approval for both uses from the Kenyan Pharmacy Board due to high efficacy and safety. Having said this, kindly allow me to make you aware of the sad reality about the presently contemplated solutions that so many are basing their hopes on, for a resolution to AIDS in Africa.

Presently constituted antiviral programs will not save Africa. Older drugs such as AZT, Lamivudine and Stavudine are no longer recommended for first line use. Depending on the status of the recipient, the death rate on these drugs ranges from 12% to 20% per year.
 However, this is not the major reason that these drugs must ultimately fail. The following realities pertain to all nucleoside analogues and cannot be ignored or glossed over:

1. Poor patient acceptance. Patient retention is under 50% within 2 years and in many cases under 25%. (As of October 2007) This is the combined effect of death, severe toxicity, and side effects leading to patient withdrawal.

2. Development of resistance to these drugs requiring extensive testing and drug change to salvage patients. This problem is beyond the capacity or financial capability of most of Africa to deal with. In addition, haphazard availability, which is common to Africa, compounds the problem of

286

resistance immensely. The death rate in patients on salvage programs remains over 20% per year in the best of circumstances.

3. The severe toxicity rate of long term usage of these drugs render them totally unacceptable from the standpoint of patient acceptance, quality of life and cost to the healthcare systems in Africa. Severe toxic reactions exceed 100% of recipients and include; anemia, neutropenia, liver failure, pancreatitis, osteonecrosis, lipodystrophy, thrombocytopenia, neuropathy, anorexia, nausea and vomiting, headache, fatigue, diarrhea, muscle pain, dizziness, insomnia, cough and the list goes on.

4. Most importantly, THESE PROGRAMS DO NOT ADDRESS THE ISSUE OF PROPHYLAXIS. No treatment program, even if successful, will succeed in the face of ever increasing numbers of infected persons, as is currently occurring.

 I know that these facts are unpleasant to any person deeply concerned about the devastation of AIDS on the African continent. However, it should be abundantly clear from a rational appraisal of the above undeniable facts that a more effective, nontoxic and lower cost solution must be implemented. Our new technology clearly meets these requirements and qualifies and can be distributed as a nutritional supplement as it contains no toxic chemicals whatsoever. Importantly organisms CANNOT develop resistance to it and this technology can be formulated as a nontoxic contraceptive vaginal gel to PREVENT TRANSMISSION OF HIV VIRUS.
In light of the above, I most respectfully request that you join with us in an effort to open a window for distribution of this modality to a cohort of patients in need of this help. This should be a relatively simple undertaking but nevertheless will lead us to the ultimate salvation of Africa.

I am sending with this letter my letter of appointment as Chief Director of Research at the Kenya Medical Research Institute as well as the letter of registration and approval of our technology by the Poisons and pharmacy Board of Republic Kenya.

I have spent over 20 years in an effort to end the AIDS epidemic in Africa and beyond, and little doubt remains that if Africa is to be saved we must work together to implement a rational program outside of traditional "business as usual" road blocks that have succeeded only in failing. Please feel free to contact me directly at any time and for any reason.

Respectfully,

Stephen D. Herman M.D. Chief Research Director, KEMRI

Not surprisingly, I am still waiting for a reply-6 months later- from anyone.

From "the HIV/AIDS epidemic in sub-Saharan Africa in a historic perspective-2006"

"In seven countries in Africa the HIV prevalence in sexually active adults exceeds 20%. By 2010-2015 the death rate will triple. Life expectancy will be reduced to 30 years. EXTENSIVE USE OF ANTIRETROVIRALS WILL NOT ALTER THE COURSE OF THE EPIDEMIC."

The future of Africa is the death of Africa - and beyond.

CHAPTER XXI
THE TALLY

In more ways than one, we have reached the final chapter. I congratulate you on having made it through to the 21st chapter as well as well as to the 21st century. I sincerely wish that I was more adept at connecting words with crystal clarity. In a world of information overload, amid a sea of conflicting opinions, truth is an elusive and difficult creature to catch.

This book did not start out to be an indictment. Unfortunately, it ended up that way. But, don't blame me-I am only the messenger. The indictment is sent down by the statements, actions and failures to act, of the perpetrators. The data is their own- not mine. In every case the studies I cite are corroborated by numerous meta- analyses from prestigious third parties - so the message is not biased by my selection.

Beyond doubt, most doctors will be incensed by what I have written here- but thousands of hours spent delving into these studies suggests the possibility that I know more about these data than they do. In other words, it will look better for them if they claim ignorance rather than admit to knowledgeable collusion.

They will most certainly accuse me of killing people by convincing patients to eschew their "life saving" medications. It is not for me to be silent, but it is for them to study their own data-and for them to do the proper science to prove beyond doubt the efficacy and safety of the products they pander for the pharmaceutical industry.

What all this has brought us to - despite their arrogance and self adulation - is a country filled with millions of autistic children and millions of demented elderly - a country with burgeoning disease of every kind - cancer, heart disease, autoimmune disease, AIDS and no real help in sight. Drugs for all the above, which work poorly, if at all, and kill more then six hundred thousand trusting patients every year.

A recent study of US college students found that an incredible 50% were suffering from either drug addiction, alcoholism or a diagnosable mental illness! Something is terribly wrong with our country and our children, and it will do little good to blame me.

The venal and felonious actions that have brought us to this state are far from over - where AIDS will go is obscure but, it is sure to be a holocaust of biblical proportions, never-the-less, it is business as usual in the medical world. The American Academy of Pediatrics now wants to put US children as young as 8 years old on statin drugs. Merck is following its lethal drug Vioxx with a next generation cox2 inhibitor ARCOXIN. The vaccine agenda is gaining momentum world wide-and the beat goes on.

At the beginning of this book I stated that legal drugs kill more than six hundred thousand people each year in America. Here is the final tally based on the data presented:

Vitamins A, C, E and antioxidants

200,000

Plavix with aspirin

75,000

Deaths as documented by JAMA

106,000

NSAIDS (including ASA)

75,000

Statin drugs leading to increased death rate

200,000

Infection due to vaccines and excessive antibiotic use [MRSA]

90,000

Total

746,000

This makes the drug industry the leading cause of death in the United States.

How many more lives would be saved if good drugs were allowed, we cannot say for sure, but, it would be substantial. Everyone will assure you that these numbers are not right and these facts are not true - but if you believe them - you haven't read this book.

Don't assume that what this book is saying is a blanket endorsement of alternative medical products. Real scientific validation is an absolute prerequisite for the recommendation of any health product. Some products in the alternative health field are good - some are not so good. But, one thing seems certain, and that is, that allopathic medicine has not stood the test of validation required to gain the confidence of America, and there is no doubt that most "alternative" drugs are far safer.

I will suggest some things you might want to consider to help fill the vacuum created by ubiquitous medical malfeasance:

Consider the following to practice a truly "healthy lifestyle".

1. Forget lowering cholesterol.
2. Forget low fat diets.
3. Eat what you like - just less of it. (Remember, fat has twice the calories of carbs and proteins). Avoid obesity.
4. Do not smoke (this is a no brainer).
5. Drink only in moderation
6. Exercise daily
7. Eat lots of fruits and vegetables
8. Remain calm
9. Avoid vaccines and be very careful what your children get.

10. Avoid all drugs when possible. (Insulin and penicillin are good drugs).
11. Treat high blood pressure only with hydrochlorthiazide (with a potassium supplement).
12. For mild analgesia use naproxen (Alleve)
13. Take calcium and vitamin D in relatively small amounts.
14. Take no supplements with vitamin A, C, or E.
15. Avoid all anti-oxidants (no matter what anybody else tells you).
16. Don't try to get too skinny - a little (overweight) doesn't hurt.
17. Above all, strengthen your immune system to slow aging and prevent degenerative changes---how?   Take ALPHAMIR daily.

Many will say that I am a disgruntled doctor with an axe to grind and you'll get no denial from me-I'm more than disgruntled- and I do have an ax to grind. I am disappointed with my medical colleagues and I do want to find a real answer to unnecessary death and suffering. If that is wrong- I plead guilty.

I wish to reiterate that I am not opposed to the use of drugs when appropriate, or the use of vaccines. I am opposed to the use of ineffective and unsafe drugs and vaccines. It is not feasible to treat the many thousands of pathogenic organisms with an endless multitude of vaccines. An alternate strategy such as the use of a safe and effective broad spectrum antiviral agent is a far more acceptable approach to this problem.

The medical profession and all doctors have a sacrosanct fiduciary duty to be more aware of the safety and efficacy of the drugs they use. They also must demand the proper and valid clinical trials required to end the controversy about the safety of vaccines. The ball is in their court.

My most profound gratitude goes to the many dedicated doctors and researchers whose honest data made this book possible and who give us hope that someday we may see an end to this inglorious era of "modern medicine."

Charles Darwin penned a cryptic message when he wrote over a drawing of the evolutionary tree of life - - **I think.**

I would like to add to that-- **I question.**

I will leave you with that pithy comment as I prepare myself for the coming onslaught.

If you have any criticism, comment, questions or would like to know more about ALPHAMIR, feel free to email me at jherman817@aol.com.